MICHEL MONTIGNAC

with a preface by Dr. Philippe ROUGER

EAT YOURSELF SLIM

OR

THE SECRETS OF NUTRITION

5th edition
entirely revised and updated
with the collaboration
of Doctor Hervé ROBERT, nutritionist
Translated from the original French version
Je mange donc je maigris !
by Daphné Jones

MONTIGNAC PUBLISHING UK

By the same author

- France : *Comment maigrir en faisant des repas d'affaires*
  Mettez un turbo dans votre assiette!
  Je mange donc je maigris!
  Recettes et Menus Montignac
  La méthode Montignac « spécial femme »
  Je cuisine Montignac Tome 1 et Tome 2
  Montignac de A à Z. Le dictionnaire de la méthode
- UK : *Dine out and lose weight*
  Eat yourself slim
  Recipes and menus
  The Montignac Method special for Women
- Spain : *Como adelgazar en comidas de negocios*
  Argentina *Las recetas de Michel Montignac*
  El método Montignac especial mujer
  Comer para adelgazar
- Italy : *Como dimagrine facendo pranzi d'affari*
  Mangio dunque dimagrisco!
- Holland : *Slank worden met zakendiners*
  Recepten en menu's Montignac
  Ik ben slank want ik eet
  Montignac van A tot Z – de Dictionaire
  Zij is slank want zij eet – Speciaal voor de vrouw
- Germany : *Essen gehen und dabei abnehmen*
  Ich esse um abzunehmen

First published in France under the title
Je mange donc je maigris! 1989.
MONTIGNAC PUBLISHING UK
108, New Bond Street
LONDON WIY9AA UK

ISBN 2-906236-41-1

PRÉFACE

When you have a weight problem to deal with, what you need above all is a pragmatic approach to it.

All too often our way of life results in gradual but inevitable weight gain, and then sooner or later obesity sets in. Being overweight has long been associated with a jovial temperament, but in fact it is more often the enemy of efficiency and the begetter of a host of ailments. So when people reach the point where they are obviously overweight, they try to reverse the process and slim down again. And then they have to decide how to tackle the problem, what " diet " to choose; or more simply, they can follow Michel Montignac's lead and take on board the notion that long-term good management of our eating is essential.

A number of methods backed by scientists prove effective in the short and middle terms, but involve such deprivation that they become restrictive and difficult to stick to... little by little comes the inevitable experience of watching the readings on the scales creep upwards again. Certainly, that was my own experience.

5

The approach advocated by Michel Montignac brings together the worlds of nutrition and gastronomy. It has the advantage that its effects are long term, provided we stick to the spirit of this new way of managing our eating. We have to change our eating habits, understand what we are eating and retrain our metabolism; in this way we can first lose weight and then remain stable at our chosen weight. The approach represents a compromise between the acceptable and the necessary. Human beings cannot be permanently restricted; they need choice, and a gastronomic approach to sensible eating.

In my own case, I found the approach attractive, especially as it worked and is still working.

Doctor Philippe ROUGER

*Maître de Conférences at the University of Paris VI
Deputy Director of the French National
Blood Transfusion Institute.*

FOREWORD

It has become commonplace to assert that we live in a society ridden with contradictions.

In the world of science we have daily evidence of the fruits of human genius and, looking at what it has been able to achieve in the last few decades, we all tend to believe that this supposed genius has unlimited potential.

But this breathtaking scientific progress is coming about unevenly. There are areas of human experience where minds are closed to all forms of progress and where sometimes our understanding even seems to take steps backwards.

Nutrition is unfortunately one of those disciplines which has been left to gather dust and where, moreover, complete anarchy appears to reign. Everyone seems to feel entitled to an opinion, the only consensus being the agreement to disagree.

And this is how things must remain for as long as the basic questions remain unanswered and no definitive theory has won general acceptance.

The " truth " in nutritional matters is nevertheless known, if only to a few privileged scientists and highly specialised members of the medical profession. But this scientifically demonstrable truth is shunned by most so-called professionals in nutrition simply through an ultra-conservative determination to cling to outdated beliefs.

The truth is hard to accept because the four concepts it depends on go against traditional beliefs. They openly question conventional wisdom and the current practices which derive from it. These four concepts are as follows :

1. *The calorie theory is misconceived.* It is a hypothesis with no scientific foundation and is illusory, in that low-calorie diets inevitably lead to failure.

2. *Poor eating habits*, and in particular the over-refining and doubtful content of some foods these days, upsets people's metabolism. This is why we have to learn to make wise choices when it comes to carbohydrates.

3. *In the same way, it is important to learn to distinguish between good and bad fats*, and to choose the good ones.

4. *Finally, we must eat a diet richer in fibre*, by turning in particular to fruit, green vegetables, pulses and wholemeal bread.

" The secrets of nutrition " amount to something like the truth of the matter, the essentials we need to understand about a subject whose importance is far greater than is generally imagined. These will be of

8

interest not only those who want to lose weight or control their weight without feeling restricted and deprived, but also — above all — those who want to discover physical vitality and their optimum level of intellectual performance.

OVERWEIGHT AND CIVILISATION

Overweight, obesity even, is a social phenomenon. It is, in a sense, a product of our civilisation.

If we observe what happens in primitive societies, we can see that overweight is generally not a problem.

Similarly, obesity is nonexistent in the animal kingdom, or at least, in animals living in their natural habitat. It is only animals domesticated by man who experience its miseries.

Paradoxically, it is in the most advanced societies that overweight is most apparent. It is as though it is an inevitable corollary to a high standard of living. And indeed, this is how the phenomenon has shown up throughout history.

Without exception, it has always been amongst the richest groups that the fattest people have been found.

What is more, plumpness has often been seen as desirable. It was the symbol of social success, as well as of good health. Fat people were always said to be " looking well ".

Today attitudes have moved on. Criteria of beauty have changed, but also we have gradually become aware of the ways in which being overweight can be bad for us.

Obesity is now considered positively dangerous, for we know it is an important risk factor for our health.

If we analyse the occurrence of obesity across the world, we are forced to conclude that it has reached its most catastrophic proportions in the United States, the richest country on earth.

Now, if we examine the way in which the Americans eat, it is not difficult to deduce that their obesity is due to their poor eating habits. What is more, the situation is growing worse with every year that passes.

Contrary to what some specialists would have you believe, obesity is not a blow dealt by the gods. Even though the origins of most obesity may be hereditary, it is nonetheless the case that they are still the consequences of poor eating habits.

Trying to tackle the question without taking on board this essential aspect of the problem amounts to dealing with the symptoms (the excess weight) while neglecting the cause. The failure of traditional nutritional theory is directly due to just such a short-sighted approach. Instead of trying to get rid of the symptoms by subjecting ourselves to starvation-level diets, we would be better employed working out why it is we put on weight. Instead of blindly following lists of ready-made menus, counting calories and weighing foodstuffs, we would do better to try to understand how our bodies work and how they go about assimilating different categories of foods.

If you are going to slim and then maintain a stable weight, it seems to me that you first need to acquire some basic knowledge. So, before you put into practice the principles of the Method laid out in this book, I suggest you go through three stages of what amounts to a real awakening of understanding.

An understanding, first of all, of how the appalling eating habits we have acquired over the last few decades have led to the progressive disruption of our metabolism. For this is the situation that is at the root of obesity and poor health.

And then, an understanding of the way in which our bodies work. This necessitates learning about the functioning of our metabolism and digestive system.

And finally, an understanding of the nature of different foods, their properties and the families of foods they belong to.

In this way you can build up solid and intelligent dietary principles, as a basis for tackling your own problem and for devising not only a workable way of managing your eating but also a workable way of stabilising your weight.

This is what I invite you to discover in the course of the chapters which follow.

INTRODUCTION

Over the last few years people have often asked me how I managed to lose weight and how I now manage to stay slim. My answer — that it is all done by eating in restaurants, on a diet of business meals — has tended to raise a smile rather than convince anyone.

You too probably find it an improbable explanation, especially if you blame your own spare tyre on the fact that your social, family or professional life involves you in a little too much good eating. At least, that is your excuse.

No doubt you have already tried out some of the innumerable dietary theories in circulation, which have long since become part of received wisdom on the subject. But you will also have noticed that the theories often contradict each other, and that they tend to produce results only fleetingly, if at all. In addition, they are mostly near-impossible to fit into a normal lifestyle. Even if you are eating at home, the rules are so restrictive that it does not take you long to grow discouraged.

So here you are, no better off than you were several years ago when it comes to tackling what we will delicately refer to as your " *unwanted pounds* ".

In the early 80s, when I was in my late thirties, my scales read 12st 12lb — almost a stone more than my ideal weight.

But then again, all things considered, that did not seem too bad for a man over six feet tall and approaching forty.

Up to then I had led a fairly conventional social and professional lifestyle and my tendency to put on weight had seemed to level off. My " overeating ", if indeed I overate at all, was only very occasional and tended to occur in a family context. When you come, as I do, from South-West France, you have been brought up to value gastronomic cuisine as part of your cultural heritage.

I had long since given up sugar, or at least, sugar in coffee. I never ate potatoes, claiming to be allergic to them, and, apart from wine, very rarely touched alcohol.

My excess stone had been acquired over a period of ten years, quite gradually. When I looked around me I felt no more overweight than the average; in fact, it seemed to me I compared quite well with other people.

Then, overnight, my professional circumstances changed. I was appointed to a new post with an international dimension at the European headquarters of the American multinational company I worked for.

From then on, much of my time was spent travelling, and the visits to the company's subsidiaries that my

responsibilities entailed making were inevitably punc-
tuated with lavish meals.

Back in Paris, my responsibility for public relations
involved me in taking mostly foreign visitors to the
best French restaurants in the capital. It was simply
a part of my job but, I have to admit, not exactly the
part I dreaded most.

But three months after taking up my new post I had
put on no less than a further stone. It has to be said
that the three-week training course I had completed in
England had done nothing to help matters either.

At any rate, alarm bells were ringing, and urgent
action was called for.

Like everyone else, I started off by trying to apply the
usual weight-loss rules and, like everyone else, I
became thoroughly disillusioned with the lack of
positive results.

But soon afterwards, as luck would have it, I came
across a general practitioner with a keen interest in
nutritional problems. He gave me some advice, and
the guidelines he suggested to me seemed to call into
question the fundamental basis of traditional dietetics.

It was not long before I was achieving very promis-
ing results. So I then decided to delve further into the
theory. This I was quite well placed to do, as I worked
for a pharmaceutical company and found it relatively
easy to come by the scientific information I needed.

Within a few weeks I had gathered together most of
the French and American papers which existed on the
subject. I already knew that certain rules brought
results, but I wanted to get to the root of the scientific
explanations, to know how and in what circumstances

the rules would work and what limits there might be to their effectiveness.

From the start I had refused to eliminate anything much from my diet, with the exception of the sugar which I had already given up. When it is your job to entertain guests in restaurants, counting calories or restricting your meal to " an apple and a hard-boiled egg " is out of the question. Some other solution had to be found.

In the event, I lost 2 stone on a daily diet of business meals, and I will explain to you later how and why it happened.

But understanding the basic principles and applying them are two different things.

After a few months, friends and colleagues were asking me to explain the Method to them, and I managed to condense the main points into three typed pages. As far as possible, I tried to spend at least an hour explaining the scientific basis to each interested individual. Sometimes this was not enough, though, and people's results were jeopardised by fundamental misunderstandings. In every case, these had arisen where the principles underlying the Method contradicted conventional wisdom. Handed-down preconceptions proved too firmly entrenched to override, and confusion resulted. Gradually I realised that there was a clear need for a more complete explanation.

So this book is intended as *a guide* and, in writing it, I have aimed to do the following :

1. To remove the mystique from some of our more entrenched ideas, and convince the reader that they deserve to be abandoned.

2. To set out the basic scientific information needed to understand how nutrition works.

3. To formulate some simple rules and explain briefly their technical and scientific basis.

4. To give detailed guidance on actually using the Method.

5. To make the book as far as possible a methodological handbook that the reader can use as a *practical reference source.*

Over the last few years, under professional guidance, I have observed, researched, tested, experimented and tried out. I am now convinced that the method of losing weight I have worked out is both effective and easy to apply.

As you read on, you will discover that *we do not put on weight because we eat too much, but because we eat badly.*

You will learn to manage your eating much as you manage your finances.

You will learn to reconcile your social, family and professional commitments with your personal pleasure in eating.

In short, you will learn how to *improve your eating habits without taking the fun out of your meals.*

This book does not set out to be a " diet book ". It suggests to you a quite new approach to eating, which allows you to *learn to control your weight while continuing to enjoy the pleasures of eating,* whether at home, with friends or in a restaurant.

And, once you adopt this new way of eating, you will be surprised to find that one result will be a long-lost feeling of physical and mental energy returning to you as if by magic. I will explain how this comes about.

You will discover that often particular eating habits are at the root of a lack of dynamism, and that this explains why you are under-performing, whether in sport or in your professional life.

You will learn how, by adopting a few fundamental and easy-to-apply nutritional principles, you can eliminate entirely the bouts of tiredness you probably suffer from and rediscover your full vitality.

This is why, even if you are only a little overweight — or not overweight at all — it is still important to understand the basis of the Method and to master the principles of good management where your eating is concerned.

It is the passport to the discovery of a new feeling of vitality, which will enable you to be more effective in both your personal and your professional life.

You will also notice that any gastro-intestinal problems you had resigned yourself to having to live with will disappear completely and permanently, because your digestive system will be properly back in balance.

You will find that in the course of this book that I sing the virtues of good French cuisine in general, and of wine and chocolate in particular. However, my intention is not to trespass upon the territory of the excellent gastronomic guides which I am sure you have on your shelves. Not that I am not tempted to do so, as I have always found it very difficult to dissociate food from pleasure, or simple cooking from gastronomic cuisine.

Over the years I have been privileged to visit some of the world's finest restaurants, and shaking hands with a great chef is to me a gesture of both respect and admiration.

Great cuisine, which is often the simplest cuisine, has become a recognised art form — an art which, personally, I would be inclined to place above all others.

CHAPTER I

THE CALORIE MYTH

The theory of slimming based on the low-calorie approach is without doubt the greatest scientific " fudge " of the twentieth century.

It is nothing more than a snare, a deception, a dangerous and simplistic hypothesis, lacking any real scientific basis. And yet it has dictated our eating habits for over half a century.

You have only to look around you to see that the more well-upholstered, plump, fat or even obese people are, the more religiously they count the calories they consume.

With very few exceptions, anything which has passed for a " diet " since the beginning of the century has essentially been based on the low-calorie theory.

How misguided can you be! No serious or long-term success can be achieved from such a method. Not to mention the side-effects, which can be devastating.

At the end of this chapter I will have more to say on the scandalous sociocultural phenomenon which has built up around the subject of calories in food. For we have reached a point where what has happened can only be described as mass brainwashing.

THE ORIGINS OF THE CALORIE THEORY

In 1930 two American doctors, Newburgh and Johnson, of the University of Michigan, suggested in one of their papers that " obesity results from a diet too high in calories, rather than from any metabolic deficiency ".

Their study on energy balance was based on very limited data and, above all, had been conducted over too short a period to deserve serious scientific acceptance.

This did not prevent their study from being immediately and widely acclaimed as irrefutable scientific truth, and it has been treated as " gospel " ever since.

A few years later, however, Newburgh and Johnson, concerned at the publicity which had been given to their discovery, somewhat hesitantly published some serious reservations they had concerning their previous findings. These went entirely unnoticed. Their initial theory was already integrated into the syllabus of most Western medical schools, and there it remains to this day.

THE CALORIE THEORY

A calorie is the amount of energy needed to raise the temperature of one gram of water from 14° to 15° centigrade.

22

The human body needs energy, first and foremost to maintain its body temperature at 98.6° Fahrenheit. But as soon as the body is active, it needs extra energy to stand vertical, to move, to speak, and so on. And on top of that yet more energy is needed to eat and digest food and carry out the basic activities of life.

The body's daily energy requirements vary according to the person's age, sex and individual needs.

The calorie theory is as follows :

If a particular individual needs 2,500 calories a day and consumes only 2,000, a 500 calorie deficit results. To compensate for the deficit, the body will draw on its fat reserves to find an equivalent amount of energy, and weight loss will result.

If, on the other hand, an individual has a daily intake of 3,500 calories when only 2,500 are needed, the excess 1,000 calories will automatically be stored as body fat.

The theory is therefore based on the assumption that there is no loss of energy. It is purely mathematical, drawn directly from Lavoisier's theory on the laws of thermodynamics.

At this point we may well be wondering how it was that prisoners in Nazi concentration camps managed to survive for almost five years on only 700 to 800 calories a day. If the calorie theory was correct, the prisoners should have died once their body fat was used up — in other words, within a few months.

Similarly, we may wonder how people with big

appetites who consume 4,000 to 5,000 calories a day are not fatter than they are (some even remain skinny). If the calorie theory was correct, these hearty eaters would come to weigh 60 to 80 stone within a few years.

Furthermore, how can you explain why some people continue to put on weight even when they reduce their daily calorie intake by eating less? Thousands of people go on gaining weight like this while starving themselves to death.

THE EXPLANATION

The first question is : when the consumption of calories is reduced, why does weight loss not follow?

Actually, weight loss does occur, but only temporarily. This is, in fact, where Newburgh and Johnson went wrong, in that they collected their data over much too short a period of time.

The phenomenon works like this :

Suppose that an individual needs 2,500 calories a day and that, over a long period, he consumes accordingly. If, suddenly, the ration of calories drops to 2,000, the body will draw on an equivalent quantity of stored fat to compensate and weight loss will be seen to occur.

However, if from now on the daily intake of calories is limited to 2,000, instead of the 2,500 previously consumed, the body's survival instinct comes into play. It quickly adjusts its energy requirements to match the level of calorie intake : if it is only given 2,000 calories, it will only use up 2,000 calories. Weight loss will quickly cease. But the body does not stop there. Its instinct for survival will lead it to take greater precautions yet, and lay down reserves for possible future need. If from now on it is supplied with 2,000 calories, it will simply reduce its energy needs to, say, 1,700 calories and store the other 300 in the form of body fat.

So this is how we end up achieving the very opposite of the result we were aiming for. Paradoxically, although the subject is eating less, he will gradually put weight back on again.

In practice, the human body, constantly driven by its survival mechanisms, behaves no differently from the starving dog which buries its bone. Despite what we might think, it is when the dog is not fed regularly that it reverts to its inborn instincts and buries its food, saving it for the day when it may otherwise go hungry.

How many of you, I wonder, have fallen victim at one time or other to this unfounded theory of balancing calories?

You will certainly have come across obese people who were actually starving themselves to death. This is especially common among women. Psychiatrists' consulting-rooms are full of women being treated for depression induced by trying to follow such a diet. They have become dependent on this vicious circle, knowing that breaking away from it will only entail putting back on more weight than they have lost.

Most members of the medical profession do not want to know. They do realise their patients are not losing weight, but they put it down to cheating and secret binges. Some slimming professionals even run group therapy sessions, at which members are applauded when they are able to show they have lost weight and made to feel ashamed of any gain.[1] The mental cruelty involved in these practices is positively mediaeval. Moreover, stipulating a 1500 calorie diet without detailing what it is to contain is quite inadequate. It simply serves to focus on the energy value of foods without taking account of their nutritional value.

Apart from a few specialists, doctors tend to be disinclined to update their understanding of these matters and are usually not knowledgable about them in the first place. Where nutrition is concerned, they seem to have little scientific understanding going beyond the commonly held views.

What is more, it is not a field in which doctors in general are particularly interested. I have noticed that of the twenty or so I have worked with on this book, all of them, without exception, were originally led to research and experiment in the field because they themselves had a serious weight problem to solve.

What is heart-rending, even scandalous, is the fact that the general public has been allowed to go on believing that the calorie theory was scientifically proven. It is sad that the theory became accepted and now constitutes one of the basic assumptions of western civilisation.

Not a week goes by without one women's magazine or another splashing an article on slimming. We are presented with the latest menus developed by some team of dieticians, based on the calorie theory and suggesting something along the lines of " a tangerine

---

1. This is particularly widespread in the United States.

for breakfast, half a rusk for elevenses, a chick-pea for lunch and an olive in the evening... "

It is amazing how the low-calorie approach has managed to delude people for so long. There are two explanations, though. One is that a low-calorie diet invariably produces a result of sorts. Lack of food, which is the basis of the method, inevitably leads to some loss of weight. But the result, as we have seen, does not last. Not only is a return to square one inevitable, but in most cases more weight is gained than is lost. The second explanation is that " low-calorie " products today constitute a sizeable market sector.

Exploitation of the theory, under the guidance of dietary " experts ", has created such a market that vested interests now have to be contended with, principally those of the food industry and a few misguided chefs.

So the calorie theory is false and now you know why. But that is not the end of it. The theory is so ingrained in your mind that for some time to come you will catch yourself still eating according to its principles.

And when we start discussing the method of eating that I am recommending to you in this book, you may well feel confused at first, because what I am suggesting seems to be completely at odds with this famous theory.

If this happens, just reread this chapter until everything is completely clear to you.

The tribulations of the under-nourished or the martyrdom of the obese

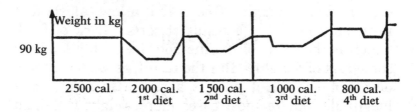

The graph above illustrates how repeated attempts at following a low-calorie diet creates resistance to weight loss.

It can be seen that the more the number of permitted calories is reduced, the less effective the diet becomes and the more liable the body is not only to revert to its original weight but also to lay down additional reserves of fat.

28

CHAPTER II

CLASSIFICATION OF FOODS

This chapter is, I think, the only one which may seem a little complicated to take in and assimilate. Bear with me if it seems rather technical; the remainder of the book, I promise you, will prove very easy to read.

Throughout the rest of the book, though, I shall be mentioning different categories of foods. If you are not familiar with these categories, you will find the Method in general hard to understand.

I have tried to reduce this chapter to its simplest, including only the information that is essential to understand what follows.

But if, despite this, you catch yourself yawning over it and are feeling drowsy by line ten or so, skip to the summary at the end of the chapter. Before you start actually trying to apply the method, though, it will be *essential* to return to the main part of the chapter, or you may not understand what you are doing.

Foods are edible substances containing a number of organic elements, such as proteins, lipids, carbohydrates, minerals and vitamins. They also contain water and non-digestible matter, such as fibre.

PROTEINS

Proteins are the organic cells that make up living matter : muscle, the various organs, including the liver and the brain, the skeletal structure, and so on. They are themselves composed of simpler elements called amino acids. Some of these are manufactured by the body, while most of the others are introduced into the body in a variety of foods. Food protein comes from two sources :

— *Animal sources :* proteins are found in large quantities in meat, fish, cheese, eggs, milk.

— *Vegetable sources :* soya, almonds, hazelnuts, whole cereals and certain pulses also contain protein.

Ideally, we should consume as much vegetable protein as animal. Protein is essential to the body :

— for building cells

— as a potential source of energy, once it has been converted into glucose (via the Krebs cycle).

— for making certain hormones and neurotransmitters [1].

— for the production of nucleic acids (essential for reproduction).

A diet deficient in protein can have serious conse-

---

1. A neurotransmitter is a chemical substance which is released by nerve cells when they are stimulated and whose function is to trigger appropriate biological activity.

quences for the body; these include muscle deterioration and wrinkling of the skin.

A child should consume about 60g of protein per day, while an adolescent needs 90g. The adult daily intake should be 1g per kilogram of body weight, subject to a minimum of 55g for women and 70g for men.

In addition, an adult's protein consumption should represent at least 20 % of the daily energy intake. If substantially too much protein is consumed, however, and physical activity is low, the excess protein will remain in the body and is converted into uric acid, which is the basic cause of gout.

With the exception of eggs, neither animal proteins nor vegetable proteins alone can achieve the necessary balance of amino acids.

The absence of one amino acid can constitute an impediment to the assimilation of others. The diet should therefore include both animal and vegetable proteins.

A vegan diet, based solely on vegetable protein, will be unbalanced, in that it will be lacking in cystine, which will result in problems with nail and hair growth.

A vegetarian diet which includes eggs and dairy produce, on the other hand, can be perfectly well balanced.

CARBOHYDRATES

Carbohydrates are molecules composed of carbon, oxygen and hydrogen.

Blood glucose level (glycaemia)

Glucose is the body's principal " fuel ". It is stored in the form of glycogen in the muscles and liver.

The blood glucose level (or blood sugar level, or glycaemia) is simply the level of glucose in the blood-stream. On an empty stomach, this is normally one gram per litre of blood.

When carbohydrates (bread, honey, starchy foods, cereals, sweets, etc.) are ingested on an empty stomach, the effect on the blood sugar level is found to be as follows :

— The first stage is that blood glucose rises (to a greater or lesser extent, according to the nature of the carbohydrate).

— The second stage is that, after insulin has been secreted by the pancreas, the blood glucose level falls and the glucose is released into the body's tissues.

— So, thirdly, the blood sugar level reverts to normal *(see graph on the following page).*

Traditionally, it was usual to place carbohydrates in one of two distinct categories, " quick sugars " and " slow sugars ", the terms referring to the body's rate of absorbing them.

" Quick sugars " were simple sugars (such as glucose) and disaccharides, such as the sucrose found in refined sugars (both cane and beet), honey and fruit.

The term " quick sugar " owed its existence to the belief that, because of the simple nature of the molecule, these sugars were rapidly absorbed by the body after ingestion.

Conversely, " slow sugars " referred to all carbohydrates whose more complex molecule had first to be chemically converted into simple sugar (glucose) in the course of digestion. This applied notably to starches, from which, it was thought, glucose was released into the body slowly and progressively.

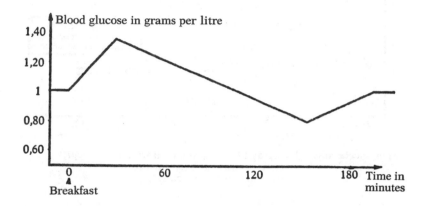

This way of classifying carbohydrates is today completely outdated, and is based on a misconceived theory.

Recent studies show that the complexity of the carbohydrate molecule does not actually determine the speed with which glucose is released and absorbed into the body.

It is now accepted that the glycaemic peak (that is, the point of maximum absorption) is reached at the same rate for any carbohydrate eaten in isolation and on an empty stomach, and occurs about half an hour after ingestion. Therefore, instead of talking about their speed of absorption, it is more to the point to consider different carbohydrates in terms of their potential to induce a greater or lesser rise in blood

33

glucose, that is, in terms of the sheer quantity of glucose they produce.

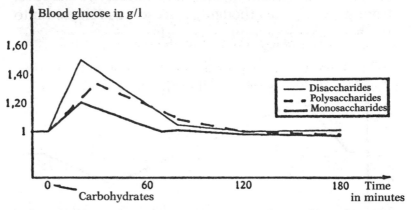

Monosaccharides (glucose and fructose found in fruit and honey)
Disaccharides (white sugar, maltose in beer, lactose in milk)
Polysaccharides (cereals, flours, potatoes, pulses)

So it is now agreed by scientists and others in the field of nutrition (see bibliography) that carbohydrates should be classified according to what is called their hyperglycaemic potential, as defined by the glycaemic index.

The glycaemic index

The potential of each carbohydrate to induce a rise in blood glucose (glycaemia) is defined by the glycaemic index, first used in 1976. This index derives from the area below the curve (shaded on the graph) of the hyperglycaemia induced by ingestion of the particular carbohydrate.

Glucose is arbitrarily given an index of 100, standing

34

for the area below its own hyperglycaemic curve. The glycaemic index of other carbohydrates can then be arrived at using the following formula :

$$\frac{\text{area below curve for the carbohydrate tested}}{\text{area below curve for glucose}} \times 100$$

The greater the hyperglycaemia induced by the carbohydrate in question, the higher will be its glycaemic index.

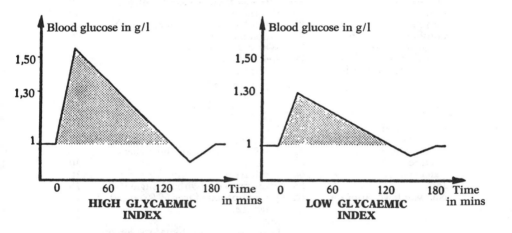

It should be noted that chemical processing of carbohydrates raises their glycaemic index. For example, cornflakes have a glycaemic index of 85, while corn (maize) in its natural state has an index of 70; instant potato has a glycaemic index of 95, whereas the index of boiled potatoes is 70.

We also know that it is both the quantity and the quality of the fibre in a carbohydrate which determines whether it has a high or low index; soft white baps have an index of 95, white baguette an index of 70, wholemeal bread 50, 100 % stoneground wholemeal bread 35, white rice 70 and wholegrain rice 50.

GLYCAEMIC INDEX TABLE

CARBOHYDRATES with high glycaemic index (bad carbohydrates)		CARBOHYDRATES with low glycaemic index (good carbohydrates)	
Maltose	110	Wholemeal bread or bread with	
Glucose	100	bran	50
Baked potatoes	95	Wholegrain rice	50
Very white bread	95	Peas	50
Mashed potatoes	90	Wholegrain cereals without sugar	50
Honey	90	Oat flakes	40
Carrots	85	Fresh fruit juice (without sugar)	40
Cornflakes, popcorn	85	Wholemeal rye bread	40
Sugar (sucrose)	75	Wholewheat pasta	40
White bread	70	Red kidney beans	40
Refined cereals with		Dried peas	35
sugar	70	100 % stoneground wholemeal	
Chocolate bars	70	bread	35
Boiled potatoes	70	Milk products	35
Biscuits	70	Dried beans	30
Corn (maize)	70	Lentils	30
White rice	70	Chickpeas	30
Brown bread	65	100 % stoneground wholewheat	
Beetroot	65	pasta	30
Bananas	60	Fresh fruit	30
Jam	55	Fruit preserve (without sugar)	25
Non-wholewheat pasta	55	Dark chocolate (over 60 % cocoa)	22
		Fructose	20
		Soya	15
		Green vegetables, tomatoes, lemon,	
		mushrooms	< 15

So, for simplicity's sake, I propose to place carbohydrates in one of two categories : " good carbohydrates " (with a low glycaemic index) and " bad carbohydrates " (with a high glycaemic index). This is the distinction which, as you will discover in the following chapters, will enable you to pinpoint, among other things, the reasons why you may be overweight.

Bad Carbohydrates

These are all the carbohydrates whose absorption leads to a large rise in blood glucose.

This applies to table sugar in whatever form (on its own or combined with other foodstuffs, as in cakes). The classification also covers all processed carbohydrates, such as white flour and white rice, and also alcohol (particularly spirits), as well as potatoes and corn (maize).

Good Carbohydrates

Unlike the carbohydrates mentioned above, " good carbohydrates " are those which are only partly absorbed by the body, and which therefore produce a much smaller rise in blood glucose level.

They include whole cereals (unrefined flour, for example), wholegrain rice and some starchy foods, such as lentils and broad beans. Most importantly, they also include most fruits, and all the vegetables which are classified as fibre (leeks, turnips, lettuce, green beans, etc.) and which all contain a small quantity of glucose.

LIPIDS (or FATS)

Lipids, or fats, have complex molecules. They are divided into two broad categories, according to their origin :

— *Lipids of animal origin :* these are found in meats, fish, butter, cheese, cream, etc.

— *Lipids of vegetable origin :* these include peanut oil, margarine, etc.

Lipids can also be divided into two categories of fatty acids :

— *Saturated fatty acids,* found in meat, cooked meats and pâtés, eggs and dairy products (milk, butter, cheese, cream).

— *Monounsaturated and polyunsaturated fatty acids ;* these are the fats that remain liquid at room temperature (sunflower oil, rapeseed oil, olive oil), though some can be solidified by hydrogenation (as in margarine manufacture). Also included in this category are all fish oils.

Lipids are necessary in the diet. They contain a number of vitamins (A,D,E,K), as well as essential fatty acids (linoleic acid and linolenic acid), and are needed for the synthesis of various hormones. Only cold pressed virgin oils can be guaranteed to retain their essential fatty acids.

When lipids are mixed with bad carbohydrates, their absorption by the body is interfered with and, as a result, a high proportion of the energy the lipids provide is stored as body fat.

As a general rule, we eat too much fat. Fried foods, doughnuts, unnecessary sauces and the use of too much fat in cooking have crept into our eating habits ; a lighter diet, avoiding excessive use of fats, need be no less delicious.

Some of the lipids are the villains in the cholesterol story, but here again, there are two types of cholesterol, " good " and " bad ". The aim should be to keep the total cholesterol level as low as possible, with " good " cholesterol accounting for as much as possible of the total.[1]

What needs to be understood is that not all lipids lead to an increase in " bad " cholesterol. In fact, some of them even tend to lower the " bad " cholesterol level significantly.

To give a complete picture, it is necessary to divide fats into three further categories :

1) *Fats which raise cholesterol*

These are the saturated fats found in meat, butter, cooked meats, cheese, lard and milk products.

2) *Fats which have very little effect on cholesterol*

These are the ones found in shellfish, eggs and skinless poultry.

3) *Fats which lower cholesterol*

These are the vegetable oils : olive oil, rapeseed oil, sunflower oil, corn oil, etc.

As for fish oils, they play no real part in cholesterol metabolism, but help prevent cardiovascular disease by bringing down the level of triglycerides and helping avoid thromboses. We ought therefore to consume oily fish (salmon, tuna, mackerel, herrings, sardines).

The weight-loss Method which I am suggesting depends in part on choosing between " good " and " bad " carbohydrates. In the same way, choices have to be made between " good " and " bad " lipids, especially if you tend to have a high cholesterol level or simply want to protect yourself permanently from the risk of it, with a view to avoiding cardiovascular

---

1. See Chapter VIII on High Blood Cholesterol.

disease[1]. Avoiding excessive consumption of saturated fats is an essential part of the Method.

DIETARY FIBRE

Dietary fibre is a substance found mainly in vegetables, pulses, fruit and whole cereals.

Although it is true that it has no actual energy value, it nevertheless plays an extremely important role in the digestive process. The cellulose, lignin, pectin and gums that it contains ensure good intestinal function, and lack of dietary fibre is the cause of most cases of constipation. Moreover, fibre is very rich in vitamins, major minerals and trace elements[2], without which serious deficiencies can occur.

It also blocks the absorption of fats, so reducing the risk of atherosclerosis.

Fibre has yet another advantage. It limits the toxic effects of certain chemical substances, such as additives and colourings. And gastro-enterologists believe that some forms of fibre have the property of protecting the colon from a number of risks, particularly that of cancer.

Over recent decades, the rise in the standard of living seen in industrialised countries has brought

---

1. A whole chapter (see page 181) is devoted to high blood cholesterol and its implications for the risk of cardiovascular disease. I urge you to pay close attention to this chapter, so as to be sure to take it into account in your choice of foods.
2. Trace elements : these are metals or similar substances present in infinitesimally small quantities in the human body and needed as catalysts for some of the chemical reactions which take place in the body.

with it a reduction in the amout of fibre consumed.

In France, for example, the current average daily consumption of fibre is 20g, whereas the recommended daily intake is 40g.

In 1925, consumption of pulses, which are particularly rich in fibre, was running at 7.3kg per person per year. Now it is down to 1.3kg.

In Italy the staple diet has always been pasta. But 30 years ago, the major part of Italians' diet consisted of vegetables (high in fibre) and wholewheat pasta — that is, pasta made with whole flour containing the wheat fibres.

SOURCES OF FIBRE
with fibre content per 100 g of food

Cereal products		Dried vegetables		Oily dried fruits	
Bran	40 g	Dried beans	25 g	Desiccated coconut	24 g
Wholemeal bread	13 g	Split peas	23 g	Dried figs	18 g
Wholemeal flour	9 g	Lentils	12 g	Almonds	14 g
Wholegrain rice	5 g	Chickpeas	2 g	Raisins	7 g
White rice	1 g			Dates	9 g
White bread	1 g			Peanuts	8 g
Green vegetables				*Fresh fruit*	
Cooked peas	12 g	Cabbage	4 g	Raspberries	8 g
Parsley	9 g	Radishes	3 g	Pears with skin	3 g
Cooked spinach	7 g	Mushrooms	2,5 g	Apples with skin	3 g
Lamb's lettuce	5 g	Carrots	2 g	Strawberries	2 g
Artichokes	4 g	Lettuce	2 g	Peaches	2 g
Leeks	4 g				

With today's higher standard of living, meat has more often than not replaced vegetables, while pasta is manufactured with refined, white flour, from which the fibre has been removed. This is the explanation given by Italian doctors for a higher incidence of obesity and also for the alarming increase in cancers of the digestive tract[1].

Furthermore, it has been shown that fibre has a beneficial effect on obesity. Introducing it into the diet has the effect of reducing both the blood glucose level and the level of insulin in the blood; as we shall see in the following chapter, it is these two factors which are responsible for the laying down of bodt fat.

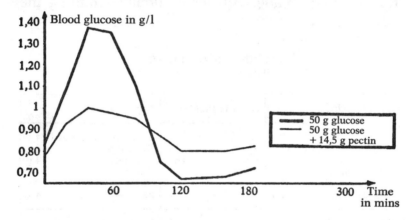

Of the four main groups of nutrients, proteins are absolutely essential to our bodies, as they contain vital amino acids which we cannot make oursel- ves. Equally important are certain lipids, which con- tain vitamins and essential fatty acids (linoleic acid and linolenic acid) that our cells are incapable of producing independently. Only carbohydrates can be

---

1. Discussed in various papers by Professor Giacosa, Head of Nutrition at the Italian National Cancer Research Centre at Genoa.

considered more expendable, since the human body is able to make its own glucose from stored fat.

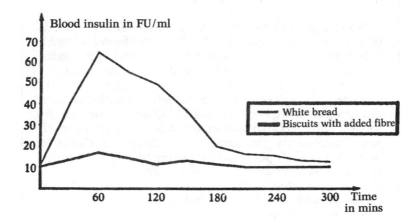

It has to be understood, though, that lipids and proteins are often found in combination in the same foods; meat is an example.

On the other hand, only carbohydrates and lipids have high energy potential.

That is why, for simplicity's sake, we will largely ignore the question of protein. So whenever we mention a particular food, we will simply put it in one of the following three categories :

— *carbohydrates (specifying whether they are " good " or " bad ")*

— *lipids*

— *dietary fibre*

When a food contains both carbohydrate and lipids, as in the case of peanuts, we will refer to it as a carbohydrate-lipid.

SUMMARY

Proteins are substances contained in a number of foods of animal or vegetable origin. They are found in meat, fish, eggs, dairy produce and pulses. Proteins are indispensable to the human body and do not make us fat.

Carbohydrates are substances that are metabolised into glucose. They occur in foods which originally contain either sugar (fruit, honey) or starch (flour, cereals, starchy foods). All carbohydrates ingested on an empty stomach are absorbed at the same rate. They are classified according to their potential for raising blood glucose; this potential is measured by the glycaemic index. It is therefore possible to draw a distinction between " good carbohydrates " with a low index and " bad carbohydrates " with a high index.

Lipids are substances which may be of either animal or vegetable origin. They are fats (meat, cooked meats, fish, butter, oil, cheeses, etc.) Some have the potential to raise blood cholesterol (meat, dairy products), while others actually help to lower it (olive oil, etc.)

Dietary fibre : in this category come all green vegetables (lettuce, chicory, leeks, spinach, French beans, etc.). Some dried vegetables, fruit and whole grains also contain a significant amount of fibre. It should be consumed frequently; failure to do so can lead to serious deficiencies.

LIST OF FOODS CLASSIFIED AS LIPIDS, CARBOHYDRATES, CARBOHYDRATE-LIPIDS OR DIETARY FIBRE

LIPIDS (1)	CARBO-HYDRATES (2)	CARBO-HYDRATE-LIPIDS	DIETARY FIBRE (3)
MEATS	FLOUR	UNSKIMMED MILK	ASPARAGUS
- LAMB	BREAD	WALNUTS	GREEN SALADS
- BEEF	RUSKS	HAZELNUTS	SPINACH
- VENISON	POTATOES	ALMONDS	TOMATOES
- VEAL	RICE	PEANUTS	AUBERGINES
- PORK	PASTA	BRAINS	COURGETTES
COOKED MEATS	SEMOLINA	LIVER	CELERY
POULTRY	TAPIOCA	SOYA FLOUR	CABBAGE
RABBIT	DRIED BEANS	WHEATGERM	CAULIFLOWER
FISH	PEAS	EGG PASTA	SAUERKRAUT
CRAB	LENTILS	CASHEWS	FRENCH BEANS
SHRIMPS	CHICKPEAS	COCONUT	LEEKS
SCAMPI	CARROTS	CHOCOLATE	ARTICHOKES
LOBSTER	SUGAR	OLIVES	PEPPERS
EGGS	HONEY	CHESTNUTS	CHICORY
BUTTER	CORN (MAIZE)	SWEET CHESTNUTS	MUSHROOMS
CHEESES	FRUIT	SCALLOPS	TURNIPS
OILS	DRIED FRUIT	OYSTERS	SALSIFI
MARGARINES		AVOCADO	FRUIT
			DRIED VEGETABLES

(1) All the foodstuffs in this column (except butter, oils and margarine) also contain protein.
(2) Some carbohydrate foods, such as pulses, also contain protein.
(3) Containing a very small amount of carbohydrate.

CHAPTER III

SO WHERE DO THOSE EXTRAS POUNDS COME FROM?

As we saw in Chapter I, an excess of " calories taken in " over " calories burned up " does not in itself explain why we put on weight. In other words, it does not account for how the body comes to store fat. There has to be some other explanation, and that is what we shall look at in this chapter.

INSULIN

Whether or not we accumulate body fat is directly linked to the secretion of insulin, so we will first take a brief look at this. *Insulin* is a hormone secreted by the pancreas[1] and it plays a vital role in human metabolism. Its function is to act on the *glucose* (i.e. the sugar) in the bloodstream in such a way that the glucose is absorbed into the body's tissues. The glu-

---

1. Insulin is a hormone secreted by small groups of cells in the pancreas called the islets of Langerhans.

cose can then either be used to satisfy the body's immediate energy needs or, if there is a surplus, it can be stored as body fat.

So let us look at a few hypothetical examples to see under what conditions and with what types of food body fat is likely to be produced, and to what extent.

INGESTING A CARBOHYDRATE

Let us take the example of a piece of bread, eaten on its own.

Bread is a carbohydrate, whose starch is broken down into glucose, which in turn passes directly into the bloodstream. The body is suddenly in a state of hyperglycaemia [1] (that is, the level of glucose in the blood is raised). The pancreas thereupon secretes *insulin* in order to :

1. release the glucose into the body tissues, either to be stored short-term as glycogen which will be used for the body's immediate needs, or to be stored for the longer term in the form of body fat.

2. lower the blood glucose level (see chapter on hypoglycaemia).

INGESTING A CARBOHYDRATE
WITH A LIPID

When, for example, you eat a piece of bread *with butter*, the metabolic process is similar to the one described in the previous paragraph.

---

1. See Chapter VI on Hypoglycaemia.

48

The carbohydrate is broken down into glucose; the blood glucose level rises; the pancreas secretes insulin.

However, there is a fundamental difference. In this example the lipid is converted into a fatty acid in the blood.

If the pancreas is in perfect condition, the quantity of insulin secreted will be exactly right for the amount of glucose to be dealt with. If, on the other hand, the pancreas is defective, the amount of insulin released may be greater than is needed to deal with the glucose. The result is that a part of the lipid's energy, which would normally simply be eliminated, will in this instance be stored as body fat. So you can now see that it is the condition of the pancreas that determines whether an individual will tend toward plumpness or will be able to eat absolutely anything without putting on an ounce : the person who puts on weight easily has a tendency to hyperinsulinism.

INGESTING A LIPID ON ITS OWN

Let us take as our example a piece of cheese, eaten *on its own.*

The metabolism of a lipid on its own involves no release of glucose into the bloodstream. Consequently, the pancreas secretes virtually no insulin.

In the absence of insulin, the energy cannot be stored away as fat.

That does not mean that ingesting the lipid has served no purpose. During the process of digestion the body extracts from it all the substances essential to its metabolism, particularly vitamins, essential fatty acids and minerals (such as calcium from milk).

This example has been deliberately simplified. Even though it is based on sound scientific principles, you may be inclined to smile at its apparent simplicity. For, as you will have guessed, the reality is somewhat more complicated.

The example does illustrate, though, the *essence* of the process we are looking at, and the essence of what we need to know in order to understand the basic rules we are going to take as our guide.

But although this chapter seems to me the most important in the book, in that it shows how body fat is created, it will not yet have explained to you how, by continuing to eat perfectly normally, but " *differently* ", you can shed all those unwanted pounds and then maintain your ideal weight.

Note : The pancreas is, in a sense, the conductor of the metabolic orchestra. If it is in good condition it will fulfil its role in bringing down the blood glucose level by secreting the appropriate amount of insulin. If it is not functioning well, if there is hyperinsulinism, it will tend to trigger the mechanisms which lay down fatty acids abnormally as body fat. So it is the pancreas, with its insulin-producing function, which turns out to be responsible for those extra pounds. However, we shall see later on that a diet with too much carbohydrate leads in the long term to pancreatic dysfunction.

CHAPTER IV

THE PRINCIPLES
OF STOCK CONTROL

In the previous chapter we concentrated on the principal mechanism by which " stocks " of body fat accumulate, answering the question " Why do we put on weight ? ".

You saw how, *when the pancreas is not functioning well, the carbohydrate-lipid combination can lead to excess weight.* In fact, though, rather than " carbohydrate ", we should perhaps say " bad carbohydrate ", because, as we saw in Chapter II, it is not so much the presence of carbohydrate but the type of carbohydrate which is at the root of the problem.

Maybe you knew this already. But you may not have known the scientific explanation of the mechanism.

And you may not have realised either how you can apply these basic principles to a *particular way of eating* which can help you reach and maintain your ideal weight.

Suppose, for example, that you are a man weighing thirteen and a half stone, and your ideal weight for your height should be eleven and a half stone. In other words, you are two stone overweight. Well, it is true that some people have an inborn tendency to above-average weight and more rounded contours, but this is the exception rather than the rule. And even if they are made that way, that does not mean that the Method will not work for them. Quite the reverse!

Like many of your contemporaries, you were probably somewhere near your ideal weight in your early twenties. But little by little, those few extra pounds crept up on you without your realising it.

The reasons for this kind of weight gain seem to be more or less the same for everyone : a more sedentary lifestyle and a change in eating habits.

The first obvious change often occurs when you get married and make changes in your social life. For women, having children can also make a difference.

But, above all, what generally sets its mark on your waistline is how you change your eating patterns in response to the demands of your professional and social life.

So, anyway, there you are a good few pounds too heavy and now you want to know what you can do about it.

Well, let us just look at the purely technical aspects of the question.

The basic principle underlying the new way of eating described here relies in part on avoiding, in general, combining lipids with bad carbohydrates. At the same time, care is taken to give preference to good lipids, so as to guard against cardiovascular disease.

Lipids will be accompanied by a variety of vegetables, notably those with a high fibre content (we will look at this in detail later).

Here are some examples of meals which contain no bad carbohydrates :

1.		
	Sardines	(good lipid + protein)
	Mushroom omelette	(lipid + fibre)
	Green salad	(fibre)
	Cheese	(lipid and protein)

2.		
	Crudités (raw vegetables)	(fibre)
	Lamb with French beans	(lipid + protein + fibre)
	Green salad	(fibre)
	Strawberries	(good carbohydrate + fibre)

3.		
	Tomato salad	(fibre)
	Tuna with aubergine	(good lipid + protein + fibre)
	Green salad	(fibre)
	Cheese	(lipid + protein)

None of these three meals contains bad carbohydrates. Of course, none of them, to conform with our Method, must be accompanied by bread. And beware of fromage frais, which contains 5g of carbohydrate per 100g. This is best eaten for breakfast or at tea-time, but avoided at the end of a meal containing lipids [1].

But let us stay with the technical explanation for a moment, to see how the weight loss occurs.

We saw in the last chapter that if the food consumed

---

1. In addition, you should preferably choose "very low fat" fromage frais and strain it (through a cheese strainer) to get rid of the whey, which contains a carbohydrate called lactose.

contained no carbohydrate, the pancreas did not secrete insulin and that, consequently, no stocks of body fat would be laid down.

Given that the body needs energy to maintain its vital functions, to keep body temperature at 98.6° Fahrenheit and make essential movements, it will draw on its fat reserves for the amount of energy it needs.

So as you continue to eat perfectly normally (consuming the necessary vitamins, minerals, and so on), the body will of its own accord reduce the fat reserves which constitute your excess weight. It will meet its needs by first burning up the previously accumulated stock.

You probably know the maxim used for stock control in business : " Last in, last out ; first in, first out. "

When bad carbohydrates are present, though, this rule of stock rotation is always violated, because, as we saw in the last chapter, in this case very short-term reserves are created to meet *immediate needs* (" Last in, first out "). If these are not used up, the surplus is then trapped as body fat and there it will remain.

If we exclude bad carbohydrates from the food ingested, the body's metabolism reverts to its basic mode of operation, which is to use its stocks of fat as a first resource to meet its energy needs.

But it has probably occurred to you to wonder what happens when the body has no fat reserves left to draw on.

When they have been completely used up, so that you are " out of stock ", when the body has virtually returned to its normal weight, it then creates a sort of

" *minimum buffer stock* ", which it will automatically keep replenished in the light of its needs.

In this way the human body, like a highly sophisticated computer, sets up an optimal management program for its stock control. This functions perfectly as long as the program is not disrupted by the presence of bad carbohydrates.

However, you should not leap to the conclusion that adopting these new eating habits means bidding farewell for ever to chips, cakes and sweets. You will be able to include bad carbohydrates in your diet in Phase II, provided you do so only occasionally. They will constitute a discrepancy in your diet which you will have to take account of in managing your overall eating pattern. We will see in the next chapter how this can be quite easily achieved.

In particular, you will see how, once your system has completely reabsorbed your fat reserves and you are moving into the phase of maintaining your ideal weight, you will be able to reintroduce a certain amount of bad carbohydrate into meals containing lipids, as long as you are *careful* and *selective* about it.

Your problem is that you are suffering from what is described medically as " *poor glucose tolerance* ". This is the one factor that distinguishes you who eat normally but " run to fat " from the next person who tucks in at every opportunity and stays as thin as a rail.

It may be that your low tolerance of sugar is attributable to hereditary factors[1], but even if this is

---

1. A study of 540 adults adopted in infancy showed that heredity was a major factor in obesity (*New England Journal of Medicine*, 23.01.1986).

so, you are also undoubtedly one of the many victims of the deplorable eating habits of the society we live in.

You are, in fact, *addicted* to bad carbohydrates, and it will take a little while for you to revert to a normal level of sensitivity to them.

It all began in your childhood, with sweet drinks, biscuits, sweets and lollipops. Not forgetting the pasta and rice — all so much easier to feed children on than pureed celery or leeks. Then there was tea-time, with white bread and butter, buns, cakes, jam and grandma's ginger-cake. Later maybe you ate school dinners or did national service — more potatoes, pasta and rice. After all, you needed something to " stand by you ". And, of course, there was bread or sugar with everything. Sugar is good for your muscles, you were told.

Then came your student days, when it was a choice between the " fodder " served in the student restaurant and take-aways or sandwiches from the fast food place on the corner. Cosy little " noshes " with friends and impromptu get-togethers in student " pads " usually turned into " carbo-feasts ".

And since you have been a working man or woman, even though the quality of your meals may have improved, you are still at the mercy of the poor eating habits of those around you.

At home, because the children like them, you eat the eternal pasta, rice and potatoes, with the occasional exotic sauce. All so quick and easy, especially as these days you can get sauce mixes which do not go lumpy.

Things are no better at work. You do not always have time to go to the staff restaurant; so much quicker and easier to have a sandwich.

And then again, productivity counts; time is of the essence and you are always short of it. So lunch-time is consumed in going to the hairdresser, or just doing the shopping. It means you can get something urgent done, but it also means you skip lunch. And as you have to keep going somehow, you drink coffee[1] — as strong as possible and with sugar, naturally... refined sugar, of course, but then it is always good for the muscles, even when they are doing no work.

Weekends bring barbecues and pub meals with friends, and traditional family lunches. Grandma down in the country does such wonderful baked potatoes it would be a crime not to eat them all up with that delicious leg of lamb.

So that is the story of how, just like the Michelin man, you acquired your very own spare tyre, an entirely useless one which is becoming more cumbersome by the minute.

And, above all, it is the story of how you became *addicted to the wrong kind of carbohydrates, the ones which release far too high a quantity of glucose.*

So the time has come to *rid yourself of the addiction* and, coincidentally, to lose your excess fat.

It is a question of somehow *raising your glucose tolerance threshold.* At the moment this is very low, which means that the moment you ingest the smallest amount of carbohydrate, especially bad carbohydrate, your pancreas gets to work manufacturing a disproportionate dose of insulin.

---

1. As we shall discover in Chapter V, coffee has the effect of stimulating insulin secretion, so aggravating sensitivity to carbohydrates.

In other words, the dose of insulin produced by your pancreas is no longer in proportion to the quantity of glucose released into the bloodstream. The excess insulin goes to work on some of the fatty acids and stores them as body fat. You are quite simply suffering from hyperinsulinism.

But the famous (or infamous) bad eating habits you have acquired or have had thrust upon you do not simply cause you to put on weight. They are also responsible for a number of physical problems you may have suffered from or are suffering from, the commonest being digestive ailments and fatigue, with all that these entail. These two consequences in particular will be examined in detail in the chapters on hypoglycaemia and digestion.

At this point, I want to issue a word of reassurance. What is novel about the principles of eating I am recommending to you is the fact that they will not hem you in without room for manoeuvre, in the way most traditional diets do.

The exact opposite is nearer the truth. As I made clear in the introduction, applying the rules laid out in the next chapter is very simple, as they are extremely straightforward and based to a refreshing degree on simple common sense.

At the beginning, when you will have to ban completely some foods or food combinations, you will find the process even easier if you normally have to eat out. At home it may be a little harder to change your routine from one day to the next, given that members of a family cannot easily be catered for individually. But once your partner sees the results you are achieving, reads this book too and realises that these new principles are sound and beneficial to everyone, including children, the whole family should come round to your views and adopt them enthusiastically.

But, as with any theory in this life, the principles are easy enough to accept; it is putting them into practice which can pose the problems. It may well be that, in your case, you were already familiar with the concepts set out in this book, but the lack of really practical guidance has deterred you from following the method effectively.

If you study the next chapter carefully, though, you will find there the key to winning the " battle of the bulge " and to getting back to a superb level of physical and mental fitness.

CHAPTER V

THE METHOD

So here we are at the heart of the matter. You may have found the previous chapters rather long, given that you are dying to discover what you actually have to do and itching to get down to applying the rules. After all, they are what will enable you to attain your goal of *losing weight and never putting it on again*, and all this while continuing to lead your normal social, professional and family life.

But I must stress, especially to any of you who felt inclined to skip some of the preceding chapters, that they are *absolutely essentialif* you are to apply the principles of the method logically and successfully. It is, indeed, vital to understand how certain mechanisms work and also to rid your head for ever of a few popular misconceptions on weight loss, such as the calorie theory.

As I have already explained, the method has two phases :

1. *the actual weight loss phase*
2. *the stable weight phase*, when you cruise along steadily, maintaining your new ideal weight.

PHASES I — WEIGHT LOSS

First and foremost, with a new undertaking — and an ambitious one at that — it is important to set yourself a clear goal.

So you should decide how many pounds you want to lose. Of course, each individual's body has its own rate of response, determined by a number of factors : gender, age, nutritional and dietary history, and heredity. This is why it is difficult to say how many pounds a week you will be able to lose. Some people may shed two pounds, others a bit less. And some people experience a dramatic weight loss at first, followed by more gradual loss. So do not worry if it takes you longer than someone else you know.

Perhaps you already have a more or less clear idea of how much you would like to lose. Many people would be happy to get rid of, say, half a stone to a stone, when really they could do with shedding twice that much. Personally, I would encourage you to aim high. After all, you are no doubt perfectionistic in your work. Why not be perfectionistic about your figure too ?

FOODS TO MONITOR CLOSELY

I know from experience that, psychologically, it is not a good idea to begin on a negative note. So I always used to try and start by emphasising to people what they were allowed to eat, and then telling them what they were not. But this really is unnecessarily tedious, since the list of what you can eat is so long that it could go on for ever. The list of what is forbidden is, by contrast, so short but so important that it is worth concentrating on that first.

SUGAR

Sugar is the hands-down, outright winner in the bad carbohydrates stakes.

It should always carry the skull and crossbones symbol, like other lethal substances. For it is indeed *a product which can be positively dangerous when consumed in large quantities* — as it unfortunately is by most people in our society, and especially by children.

Elsewhere I have devoted a whole chapter to sugar, so that you can be convinced once and for all of its evil role in our diet and of its nefarious consequences, not only in terms of excess weight, but also — and most importantly — because it is implicated in chronic fatigue, diabetes, gastritis, ulcers, dental caries and heart disease.

You may think it is impossible to do without sugar. Well, it is not. The proof is that for tens of thousands of years human beings did not have such a thing, and they were none the worse for that. Just the opposite, in fact.

Less than 200 years ago, sugar was still a luxury hardly ever available to most of the population. Today it does as much harm as alcohol and drugs put together.

But, you ask, if you cut out sugar completely, how do

you maintain the essential minimum of glucose in your bloodstream ?

A good question !

The answer is that the body does not need to get sugar from outside (this is just what upsets the blood glucose level). It can produce its own sugar in the form of glucose when it needs it, and this is far and away what it prefers to do. Glucose is, of course, the body's only fuel.

The body determines how much glucose it needs as it goes along, and as it does so, body fat is simply converted into the glucose needed.

So no more sugar ! You can take one of two courses ; either do without (with my full approval) or replace it with an artificial sweetener[1].

BREAD

Bread could have taken a whole chapter to itself, there are so many things that could be said about it. Good things, if we are talking about " good bread ", so rare a commodity these days, but especially bad things when it comes to the unsatisfactory product being sold by most bakeries.

Ordinary bread, being made with refined flour, is totally devoid of anything of use to the normal human metabolism. Nutritionally, its only contribution is energy in the form of starch.

From the digestive point of view, it means nothing

---

1. See Chapter IX on Sugar.

but trouble, given that all the elements which would ensure it was well digested have been removed in the course of refining the flour.

Moreover, the whiter the bread is, the " worse " it is, since its whiteness is the result of the flour being very heavily refined.

Wholemeal bread[1], and especially 100 % stoneground wholemeal bread, are much more acceptable, being made in the old-fashioned way with unrefined flours containing fibre. They release notably less glucose than white bread and are therefore less " fattening ".

But good though they are, even these types of bread will temporarily be ruled out, at least with main meals. You should, however, eat them normally at breakfast. We will look at this in detail a little later on.

If you are worried about giving up bread, let me reassure you right away.

If, in common with 95 % of the population, you consume ordinary white bread, you have nothing to lose but your excess pounds by giving it up. On the contrary, you have everything to gain from such a wise decision, refined flour being so bad for your health.

On the other hand, if you normally eat *only* stoneground or other wholemeal bread, made with unrefined flour (which shows you already have some good eating habits), you may lose the advantages of the fibre in giving it up.

But rest assured, not only can you go on eating it for

---

1. 100g of wholemeal bread contains 90mg of magnesium, whereas 100g of ordinary bread contains only 25mg.

breakfast, but we shall also be recommending that you consume fibre-containing vegetables, which are of as much, if not more, benefit for good intestinal function.

STARCHY FOODS

By starchy foods I mean floury foods containing starch. Most such foods are bad carbohydrates and some need to be completely excluded from your diet.

Potatoes

The number one starchy food is the potato. You may be interested to know that when the potato was brought back from the New World by explorers in 1540, the French firmly rejected it, considering this root vegetable fit only for pigs. They thought it so unpleasant they refused to eat it, unlike some northern European peoples, such as the Germans, the Scandinavians and the Irish, who took to it readily. It has to be said that some of these people had relatively little choice, often having not much else to eat.

For two centuries the French continued to pour scorn on the " pig root ". It was not until 1789, when Parmentier published his *Treatise on the cultivation and uses of the potato*, that people in France finally came round to eating it. The famine that was raging at the time was an additional incentive.

It was later discovered that the potato is rich in vitamins and minerals, though it loses most of these when it is cooked and, especially, when it is peeled.

66

Recent tests have shown that the potato releases a very large quantity of glucose into the system.

Traditional nutritionists generally classed the potato as a " slow sugar ", but this is mistaken. Compared to the glycaemic index of 100 of pure glucose, the boiled potato has been shown to have a glycaemic index of 70, which makes it a bad carbohydrate. Moreover, it has also been demonstrated that the method of cooking potato changes the structure of its molecule, which can make matters worse : mashed potato has an index of 90, while baking potatoes in the oven causes their index to shoot up to 95 !

So you can look upon the steaming potato on your neighbour's plate with the utmost contempt !

And remember, chips are potatoes too. (I can feel your resolution beginning to weaken !)

Chips are a carbohydrate-lipid food, rather like buttered bread. They simply cannot be eaten without the risk of putting on weight, since the oil used in the frying can be laid down as body fat.

So think of steak and chips as an absolute heresy ! Do not let the thought of this worst of all possible dietary combinations even cross your mind ! The lipid from the meat and the bad carbohydrate from the chips constitute a mixture which goes against nature.

I know the cost of foregoing this favourite meal, but it is the price to be paid for reaching your goal. When you hit your target weight, you will have no regrets about the sacrifice.

What is more, chips are frequently fried in fats which are very high in saturated fatty acids, consumption of which constitutes a significant risk factor for cardiovascular disease.

However, once or twice a year I eat chips : not because I give in when confronted with a plateful, but because I make a conscious decision to eat them (when you are no longer trying to lose weight, you can afford to make this kind of decision). But I do not eat just any chips. If you are going to indulge in a dietary discrepancy, you may as well savour it to the full and choose the best to be had. And for maximum damage limitation, accompany your chips with a green salad. Not only is it delicious, but the fibre in the salad tends to trap the starch, turning the combination into a carbohydrate which releases a more limited quantity of glucose.

When you order meat in a restaurant, get into the habit of asking what is served with it. There is always an alternative to potatoes. You can ask for French beans, tomato, spinach, aubergines, celery, cauliflower, courgettes. And if, unfortunately, there are only bad carbohydrates to choose from, then order a side-salad.

At home, when it comes to deciding what to serve with meat, adopt the same principle.

Dried beans

Some of you will no doubt be expecting me to condemn beans out of hand, given what I have just said about potato. Well, you will be wrong!

In the first edition of this book, it is true, I spared neither the bean nor that noblest of dishes in which it features, the cassoulet.

68

I now make amends for my hastiness. I have since discovered, to my surprise and great satisfaction, the virtues of the haricot bean. From now on, it must be classed as a good carbohydrate by virtue of its very low glycaemic index [1].

In addition, it is high in vegetable fibre (particularly soluble fibres) and in minerals.

So it is possible to eat beans in Phase I in the course of a protein-lipid meal.

Rice

Wholegrain rice, as it is traditionally consumed in Asia, is an entire food in itself, containing all the nutritional elements essential to life.

The white rice generally eaten these days, however, is heavily refined, to the extent that it retains hardly any nutrients, except starch, the one thing we could well do without.

Ordinary refined rice must therefore be excluded since, just like refined flour, it constitutes a bad carbohydrate with high release of glucose [2].

Wholegrain rice, on the other hand, or — even better — Canadian wild rice, can be eaten, as long as it is not mixed with lipids, such as butter or cheese. Served with tomatoes (reduced by cooking) and onions, it can make a complete dish to be enjoyed by the whole family (see Appendix 4 for recipe).

It is a great pity it is so difficult to find wholegrain

---

1. See Chapter II.
2. Release of glucose relative to an index of 100 :
Refined rice : index 70
Wholegrain rice : index 50

rice in restaurants, but this may be due to its slightly unappealing grey-brown colour.

Corn (Maize)

Maize has been cultivated for centuries, but has only been eaten by human beings for a few decades.

Forty years ago, not a tin of sweetcorn was to be found in Europe, where maize was grown exclusively as an animal feed.

In the United States, too, it was used to fatten cattle until the drought of 1929 decimated herds and ruined farmers in the Midwest. Faced with the real famine which ensued, the hungry population no longer had beef available, so decided to eat the cattle feed, or what was left of it.

And that is how America took to eating " corn ", a habit which was exported to Europe in the 40s with the post-war American occupation.

So we should not now be surprised to discover that maize has a high glycaemic index, given that for centuries it was used to fatten up cattle. But it is interesting to note that processing maize pushes up its glycaemic index still further, giving products like popcorn and cornflakes very high glycaemic potential indeed. So they are extremely fattening. In addition, processed maize contains a substance which destroys niacin; this is a vitamin necessary for growth, and lack of it can also cause metabolic imbalances and abnormal fatigue.

Pasta

Non-wholewheat pasta is by definition a bad carbohydrate, being made from refined flour, to which are added lipids such as butter, eggs, cheese and oil. And despite anything the advertising slogans may say to the contrary, the "richer" the pasta, the more it constitutes a carbohydrate-lipid and goes against our eating rules.

I admit it is a bitter blow to have to give up pasta, because there is nothing more delicious when it is fresh and well made.

However, if you have the misfortune to be served fresh non-wholewheat pasta (pasta not freshly made is not even worth considering), summon up your determination and refuse to eat it while you are in Phase I, the weight-loss phase. When you are cruising along in Phase II, have some if you think it is worth the sacrifice.

As for wholewheat pasta, and especially stoneground wholewheat pasta, made from unrefined flour, this can be included in dishes in Phase I in the course of a carbohydrate meal.

Accompanied by a tomato coulis or a basil sauce, it can constitute a meal in itself.

Indeed, wholewheat pasta is classed as a good carbohydrate, having a glycaemic index of only 45.

Other bad carbohydrates

I have deliberately discussed in greatest detail the bad carbohydrates you are most likely to be eating on a regular basis, and which you will have to give up, at least temporarily.

Other bad carbohydrates tend to be foods which contain a good deal of carbohydrate but very little protein, and which have only poor quality fibre.

The combination of these factors confers on such foods a high glycaemic index.

It is worth mentioning carrots and beetroot in this category. Also to be included are all the carbohydrate-lipid items, such as biscuits, croissants and pastries, which should be ruled out in Phase I.

Dark chocolate, if it is the bitter kind with a high cocoa content, has a low glycaemic index. However, it should be eaten only very exceptionally during Phase I, as it too constitutes a carbohydrate-lipid.

There is one more rather special kind of carbohydrate we now need to look at : fruit.

FRUIT

Fruit is a sacred subject. I know if I was tactless enough to advise you to exclude it from your diet, a good many of you would shut the book forthwith, scandalised at the mere suggestion.

For fruit has a symbolic value in our culture. It stands for life, health, prosperity. It is, first and foremost, a source of vitamins — at least, that is what we believe. Well, first let me set your mind at rest; we are not going to exclude fruit. But it is a question of learning to eat it in a different way, if we are to enjoy all its benefits without also suffering its drawbacks, such as a bloated abdomen.

Fruit contains carbohydrates (glucose, sucrose and especially fructose), but it also has fibre, which lowers its glycaemic index and reduces the amount of sugar absorbed by the body.

72

Apples and pears are particularly rich in pectin (a soluble fibre), which limits the rise in blood glucose.

Energy provided by fruit can be used rapidly by muscles and is therefore less likely to be stored and to lead to the accumulation of body fat.

This point is not relevant just to the weight-loss question which we are concerned with. It is based on the chemistry of digestion. When fruit is eaten with other items, it interferes with the digestion of those items, while itself losing most of the properties (vitamins and so on) for which it has been consumed. This is why eating fruit at the end of a meal is the biggest mistake you can make.

I know that you are probably viewing this notion with considerable scepticism, so I will explain it a little here and now, even though these points really belong in another part of the book.

For starch to be digested, it is *essential* that an enzyme called ptyalin is present. This is secreted in the saliva. Most fruits have the effect of destroying ptyalin, with the result that any starch consumed along with fruit cannot be digested. The food bolus remains " in limbo " in the stomach, where the warmth and humidity will cause it to ferment. Bloating, flatulence and indigestion can often be attributed directly to this phenomenon. Maybe this explanation sheds a little light on these familiar symptoms.

Let us now consider what happens when fruit is consumed with protein-lipids, such as meat or cheese. Fruit requires rapid passage into the intestine, where it is normally digested, but in this instance its journey is interrupted for a while in the stomach. For meat remains for some time in the stomach, where the essential enzymes account for the most important stage of its digestion.

The fruit is therefore also trapped in the stomach, where once again the effect of the warmth and humidity causes fermentation, even producing alcohol, and the whole digestive process is upset.

At the same time not only does the fruit loses all its vitamins, but (problems never come singly) the protein metabolism is also upset, and the abnormal decomposition of the proteins results in abdominal bloating.

So fruit must always be eaten on its own! That rule should be taught in schools. If it were, children would have fewer stomach upsets. It has to be said, of course, that at their age the body has the capacity to compensate for errors; but for an adult, and especially for an older person, fruit at the end of a meal is *nothing short of poisonous.*

So then when can we eat fruit?

At any time, on an empty stomach. In the morning, for example, before breakfast. But you will then need to wait about 20 minutes before starting your breakfast. You can then eat a carbohydrate-protein breakfast (wholemeal bread, cereals, skimmed milk).

It is preferable not to eat lipids after fruit. The small amount of insulin triggered by the fruit could lead the body to store the fats in the ham, eggs, bacon or cheese you might eat for a protein-lipid breakfast.

You could also eat fruit last thing at night before bed-time. It would need to be at least two to three hours after your evening meal.

For those who suffer from insomnia (which ought in any case to be partly cured by following the Method suggested in this book), it is not a good idea to consume oranges just before bed, as vitamin C can act as a stimulant.

Fruit can also be eaten in the late afternoon, provided it is well after the mid-day meal (about three hours) and at least an hour before any evening meal.

You can even eat a meal consisting entirely of fruit, as long as you really do eat nothing else.

As lemon has virtually no sugar, lemon juice (unsweetened) can be drunk at any time or used freely in seasoning (with fish or in salad dressings, for example).

Melon as a starter should also be avoided, though, as it prompts just enough secretion of insulin to trap the lipids contained in the main course.

I should like to make one last observation on the subject of fruit. Whenever possible, leave its skin on. The skin contains most of the fibre which is valuable for intestinal function, and in some cases most of the vitamins too.

Eating fruit skin and all reduces its glycaemic potential, too, so you will lose more weight (or put on less) if you follow this rule.

Among the foods to be monitored closely, there remains to be considered the question of drinks and, chief amongst them, alcohol.

ALCOHOL

Alcohol is fattening! That is what you believe, because that is what you have been told. You may even have been made to feel guilty by people who have implied that all your unwanted pounds could be put down to alcohol, with no need to look further. Let us try and make an objective assessment.

It is true that alcohol is fattening. But *much less* fattening than sugar, white bread, potatoes or rice. That is why, very soon after you have shed your unwanted pounds, you will be able to reintroduce wine into your diet in reasonable quantity (up to about half a litre of wine a day, about three glasses, for a man, though women should reduce this by a third). The energy provided by alcohol is used by the body as a first resource for immediate needs, and while the body is using this fuel it will not be burning up stored body fat. This means that the alcohol is preventing you losing weight. However, this happens in particular when it is imbibed on an empty stomach. When the stomach is already full, particularly if it is full of protein-lipids (such as meat, fish or cheese), the alcohol is metabolised much less rapidly because it is mixed with these other foods, and so produces little stored fat.

What must be categorically given up is the apéritif. If you really feel you have to keep your guests company, have something non-alcoholic like tomato juice or mineral water.

The only noble apéritif, to my mind, is a glass of good champagne or good white wine (I say " white " advisedly). But, I implore you, do not let people adulterate your wine, as often happens to disguise its mediocre quality, with blackcurrant liqueur or those other weird syrups which people come up with just for the sake of something new.

So, if you really must, accept a glass of champagne

but, above all, *do not drink it on an empty stomach.* Help yourself to a few " nibles " first.

Beware, though! They must be non-carbohydrate " nibbles ". You will soon learn to recognise them.

Crisps and cocktail biscuits of all sorts are out. Olives, cheese, cocktail sausages or fish are acceptable.

In Phase I, though, you should try to exclude apéritifs completely. Phase I is the time for being really strict in applying the basic rules of the Method, as this is the way you will lose weight.

AFTER DINNER DRINKS

Cross these off your list too. Cognac, armagnac and many liqueurs are delicious, and may be an excellent thing for the French balance of payments, but they will do nothing to improve your waistline.

Maybe you think that such drinks (known as " digestifs " in France) will help you digest your meal. Well, rest assured, once you have mastered the eating habits advocated in this book, you will have no indigestion to worry about, even after the most copious of meals.

BEER

I am not going to be much kinder about beer. In my view, it is a drink to be consumed in the strictest moderation.

Just as you may know skinny people who incessantly stuff themselves with bad carbohydrates with no ill effect, you have probably also met heavy beer drinkers with stomachs as flat as a pancake. (The wife of one of my best friends falls into this category.)

You do not need to have visited Germany to know about the usual side-effects of beer drinking, though : bloating, weight gain, bad breath and indigestion, all of which occur despite the presence of diastases (small enzymes whose function is to aid digestion). Let us just say that without diastases the consequences of beer drinking would be catastrophic.

Beer contains everything that is bad for you : alcohol (albeit in moderate quantities), gas and, above all, a large amount (4g per litre) of a carbohydrate called maltose, whose glycaemic index is 110, higher even than that of glucose. Furthermore, the combination of alcohol and sugar tends to lead to hypoglycaemia, and therefore tiredness and under-performance (see chapter on hypoglycaemia). So it is a drink with high energy potential, which means a high potential for creating stored fat.

You should give up beer, especially between meals. If you really cannot resist it, consider beer in the same way you consider chips. Indulge yourself once or twice a year, by having a pint or two of the best beer your local can provide, but make sure you choose a quality brew.

In Phase I, I would advise you to drink no beer at all. In Phase II, though, just as you can reintroduce wine in moderation, so you can, from time to time, enjoy a small quantity (33 centilitres at most) of beer with a meal.

WINE

I have left wine until last, it being the only alcoholic drink I am not entirely against.

I shall make no distinction between red and white wine, except to say that red wine generally contains more tannin. Tannin possesses particular therapeutic properties; in particular, the procyanidin it contains helps prevent atherosclerosis, with the polyphenols also present in it having a protective effect on the artery walls.

It is only a short step from this statement to the assertions of many scientists, including Professor Masquelier, that wines rich in tannin contribute to some extent to the prevention of cardiovascular disease[1].

A highly reputable medical survey, carried out in Britain in 1979 and bringing together evidence from eighteen countries, concluded that the death rate from heart attacks was lowest in populations which habitually drank wine (three to five times lower in France and Italy than in Northern European countries).

So, following our Method, wine can form a part of a normal diet, as long as reasonable limits are observed (about half a litre a day for a man, but only two thirds of this for a woman), and as long as it is consumed as late in the meal as possible, once the stomach is full of food.

In Phase I it is as well to stay away from wine if

---

1. See Dr. Maury's book, *La médecine par le vin*, published by Artulen.

possible.   In Phase II it can be drunk on a daily basis without affecting your weight.   However, wine consumption will need to be juggled carefully with other carbohydrate intake.   I am thinking in particular of chocolate and desserts in general.   But that will be the subject of a paragraph further on.

While you are in Phase I, the stage where you need to be very strict with yourself, it may prove difficult to enjoy a family occasion or a meal with friends without touching a single drop of wine.   If you suddenly announce you are not drinking, others may feel awkward about it.

My tip is to allow your glass to be filled and to pick it up as often as you would if you were drinking normally.   But just wet your lips with the wine rather than actually drinking any.

I used this trick over several weeks and I assure you that no-one ever noticed I was not drinking.

In the same way, no-one has ever noticed that I am not eating a crumb of bread.   To keep up the pretence, I always take my piece of bread and break it, but it stays beside me uneaten.

Vinegar contains only a negligible amount of alcohol, so it can be used to season crudités and salads, unless, of course, you prefer lemon.

COFFEE

Really strong coffee, Italian espresso with a caffeine content that would waken the dead, is out.   Drink decaffeinated or weak arabica coffee, which contains much less caffeine.   Decaffeinated coffee can be found everywhere these days and it is usually good. At home, too, you can make a very good decaffeinated brew. Even serious coffee drinkers cannot tell the difference.

If you are a heavy drinker of very strong coffee, it is probably because you feel the need for a stimulant to wake you up.

If you regularly " run out of steam " round about eleven o'clock or in mid-afternoon, this is because you are hypoglycaemic (see the chapter on this subject).

Caffeine is not permitted here because, although it is not a carbohydrate, it has the effect of stimulating the pancreas into producing insulin. If you have just finished a meal with no bad carbohydrates, and all surplus energy is being accounted for, it would be silly to undo the good work by drinking a cup of strong coffee and prompting the pancreas into secreting insulin which will set the fat accumulation process going. If you are a coffee drinker, you should have no difficulty in going over to the decaffeinated variety when you start applying the Method. You will soon find yourself not even feeling the need for coffee.

It is important to stress, in any case, that coffee drinkers (whether they drink coffee with or without caffeine) are laying themselves open to a further risk : that of a raised blood cholesterol level (see chapter on high blood cholesterol).

Beware of tea, too, as it can have as much caffeine as a cup of coffee and, in addition, contains tannins which can inhibit the absorption of iron !

SOFT DRINKS

These are usually based on synthetic fruit or plant extracts and all have the same major failing : they contain a great deal of sugar.

Damned by this fact, they should be excluded entirely from your diet, not only because they have a very high sugar content, but also because the artificial gases they contain lead to stomach irritation, gastritis and burping.

You should be wary of fizzy drinks, which may still be toxic even if they are based on natural extracts. Significant traces of toxins such as terpenes are frequently to be found in natural citrus fruit extracts.

The worst soft drinks are colas. If they cannot be banned, they should, like cigarettes, carry a government health warning.

At all events, it is regrettable that the consumption of colas has taken such a hold in Europe. In the words of Dr. Emile-Gaston Peeters [1],

" At the present time, cola drinks available on the European market contain about 21mg of caffeine and 102mg of phosphoric acid per 19cl (the average content of a small bottle). The caffeine is a stimulant. The high concentration of phosphoric acid can upset the calcium-phosphorus balance in the diet, leading to a serious calcium deficiency in the bones. One also needs to be sure that the phosphoric acid used does not contain a harmful level of toxic heavy metals. The conclusion is straightforward : *children and adolescents*

---

1. *Le guide de la diététique*, published by Marabout.

82

should be firmly discouraged from drinking colas. They
do no good to anyone. "

This comment speaks for itself.

So whether we are talking about your children or
yourself, the advice remains firmly the same : no
lemonade, no fizzy drinks, no cola !

MILK

Full-cream milk is a carbohydrate-lipid food; in
other words, it contains both fat and carbohydrate. It
is therefore better avoided, and skimmed milk used
instead.

The carbohydrates are found in the whey. This is
discarded in the cheese-making process, leaving only
lipids and proteins in the cheese. (There are some
exceptions to this, such as cantal and goats' cheeses.)

In " very low fat " fromage frais there remains
virtually only protein and a small amount of carbohydrate (5g per 100g).

FRUIT JUICES

I will not deal with the problems of fruit juices at
any length, because my general comments on fruit
hold good, as you might imagine, for fruit juices. They are carbohydrates and should be treated as
such.

I would advise you, however, to choose fruit rather
than fruit juice, so as to retain the full benefit of the
fibre contained in the pulp. Obviously, only home-

made fruit juice squeezed from fresh fruit is acceptable. Never drink the commercially available pseudo-fruit juices, which are devoid of vitamins and over-acidic, and to which sugar is routinely added.

PUTTING THE METHOD INTO PRACTICE
PHASE I — WEIGHT LOSS

Phase I of our Method is not all that hard to apply, as it simply consists of eliminating certain foodstuffs from your diet. But for complete success it is important that you should have a full understanding of the *basic principles* underlying what you are doing.

In my own experience, this is where some people fail. I am not for a moment casting doubt on your intellectual ability to accept new concepts. But in this case the hard part is to rid your mind completely of preconceived ideas, many of which are deeply rooted in our culture and therefore in your subconscious. The ideas presented in this book, although quite straightforward and based on the findings of doctors and researchers[1], have unfortunately not yet broken through the barriers of general acceptance. So you cannot necessarily rely on those around you for encouragement in your undertaking.

It is vital not to skip a meal. If you do, your metabolism is thrown off course and at the next meal will do its best to lay down some fat reserves. So you should have three meals a day, plus a tea-time snack if

---

1. See Bibliography.

84

you like. Avoid having an almost nonexistent breakfast and lunch, and then trying to compensate by
eating an enormous meal in the evening.

BREAKFAST

Breakfast number 1 :

This is a carbohydrate breakfast, and should contain
a significant amount of fibre.

— **Option 1 :** high-fibre bread (this means
wholemeal bread containing bran or, even better,
100 % stoneground wholemeal bread).

Nowadays in Britain, if you ask for a wholemeal loaf,
you should get one made entirely from wholewheat
flour. Wholewheat, or wholemeal (it means the same)
flours contain the whole of the product derived from
milling : the endosperm (mainly carbohydrate), the
bran (fibre, vitamin B and protein) and the wheatgerm
(rich in nutrients, such as vitamins B and E, iron and
essential unsaturated fat). The whole grain contains
up to 24 different nutrients.

Stoneground wholemeal flour has the additional
advantage that, being ground between millstones in
the old-fashioned way rather than by using modern
rollers, the wheatgerm oil is evenly distributed
through the flour. This enables the various nutrients
to work together effectively. Stoneground flour lost
favour with the milling industry in the last century, as
it cannot be stored for long periods, going rancid in a
matter of months.

Modern steel roller mills solve the problem by splitting the grain before milling and separating it into its three parts. White flours, consisting only of the starchy endosperm, have indefinite storage life because the wheatgerm has been removed. Since this means most of the essential nutrients have also been removed, the white flours we consume today contain a vast range of additives which attempt to compensate.

Bread labelled " wheatmeal " in Britain is not wholemeal; it is paler because up to 20 % of the bran has been removed. And " brown " bread is usually made from white flour, with caramel added to give a " healthy " colour. Beware, too, of bread " with added bran " : bran would not need to be added if it had not first been removed.

I advise you to choose 100 % stoneground wholemeal bread; it is not hard to find. The fact that it retains all the benefits of the wheatgerm makes it a " good " carbohydrate, with a low glycaemic index. It is rich in protein, minerals, trace elements and B complex vitamins.

You can also buy German breads (Schwartzbrot or Pumpernickel) in the larger supermarkets, but take a good look at the ingredients because they often contain sugar and, particularly, fats.

For variety, you can also eat wasa-type crispbread, made from oats.

At all events, you should rule out all forms of " biscotte ", which are likely to contain fats and often sugar.

Now, what are you going to spread on your wholemeal bread, or whatever you are eating instead? In Phase I, unlike Phase II, butter and margarine are, of course, outlawed. Equally, honey is out of the question, as is ordinary jam, which is 65 % sugar. I would suggest two possibilities :

1) a sugar-free fruit preserve, i.e. pulped fruit set with apple pectin and guaranteed to contain no added sugar. Even though it may taste similar, if less sweet, this bears no real resemblance to ordinary jam.

Since this product has a very low glycaemic index, it makes an excellent spread to go with wholemeal bread.

2) " very low fat " fromage frais or a " very low fat " yogurt. This can be eaten as it is or flavoured with a little salt or some of the preserve described above.

— Option 2 :

A Phase I breakfast can also consist of wholegrain cereals. The utmost care is needed when buying these, as they must be free of sugar, honey, caramel, rice and corn. Muesli which meets these criteria is also acceptable.

Whole cereals (including oat flakes, mixed cereal flakes and muesli) can be consumed with hot or cold skimmed milk, or mixed with " very low fat " fromage frais or " very low fat " yogurt. A little sugar-free fruit preserve can be added if need be.

In any case, avoid breakfast cereals based on white rice or corn. This rules out cornflakes, which, as we have discussed, have a glycaemic index of 85.

Bran breakfast cereals can be included, as they are very high in fibre, but make sure they are completely sugar-free.

Breakfast number 2

Breakfast number 2 is a savoury meal, based on protein-lipids, which could be ham, bacon, cheese or eggs (scrambled, boiled or fried). This is rather like a traditional British breakfast, except that in Phase I it must contain absolutely no carbohydrate. So toast and fried bread are out, even if the bread is wholemeal.

This is an ideal breakfast if you are staying in a hotel where they do not have wholemeal bread or whole cereals, or at home at the weekend when you have a little more time available.

It should, however, be the exception rather than the rule, as this type of breakfast is very high in saturated fats.

Indeed, if you have high blood cholesterol or any sort of cardiovascular disease, this meal is definitely not for you at all.

As this breakfast contains no carbohydrate at all, you will need to keep that in mind when choosing what to eat later in the day, or over a period of several days.

It is even possible to finish this protein-lipid breakfast off with a full-cream fromage frais or yogurt, but be careful not to eat more than 50g, as these products do contain a small amount of carbohydrate in the form of lactose from the milk.

What to drink at breakfast

Whichever breakfast option you choose, you can drink any of the following :
— decaffeinated coffee

— weak tea (strong tea can be just as bad as coffee)
— chicory (on its own or mixed with the coffee)
— cocoa
— skimmed milk (the powdered sort can be made up to a more concentrated mix, if you prefer).

In Phase I you should avoid chocolate drinks in general. The possible exception to this is for children, but be careful to choose a low-fat one without added sugar (such as Van Houten).

All these drinks are, of course, consumed without sugar. If you must, you can add an artificial sweetener, such as aspartame, but try to wean yourself off it over a period, so that you learn to do without sweet things.

LUNCH

Whether you eat out or at home, this meal will consist of protein-lipids, though this does not mean it need have a high fat content (see Chapter II on " good " and " bad " lipids). I will give you a few examples so you can be sure you are not making any mistakes. But my best advice is to keep consulting the list of carbohydrate-free foods in Appendix I. I would even suggest you photocopy it before you start and keep it handy. But you will soon know it by heart.

A typical lunch menu will be as follows :

A starter of crudités (raw vegetables)
Fish and/or meat
Permitted vegetables (see list)
Salad

Cheese
To drink : still water

Starters

Any kind of salad is in order, as long as none of its ingredients contains carbohydrate. This can happen if, for example, you order a salade niçoise. So, before you order anything, take the precaution of checking that it contains *no potato, corn, carrot or beetroot.*

Crudités can be seasoned with oil (preferably olive oil) and vinegar or lemon.

In Phase I you should also avoid carbohydrate-lipids, such as walnuts. If you are in a restaurant, do not order walnut salad, though a salad containing little bacon pieces will be fine. But specify that you do not want croutons; a number of restaurants have an infuriating mania for sticking them in everything!

Be on your guard! Do not let " little mistakes " (which are actually very big ones) creep in and spoil your chances of attaining your objective. Be strict with waiters and waitresses; if you have said " *without croutons* " or " *without sweetcorn* ", do not accept a mistake just because the staff are busy.

If you want to be taken at your word, you must insist that *on no condition must you find the least trace in your meal of the item you do not want.*

My own experience is that you are most likely to be successful in this if you claim to be allergic to the item. It works every time. Anyway, as long as your starter contains only things like French beans, leeks, cabbage, cauliflower, tomato, chicory, asparagus,

90

mushrooms, radishes, cheese or cooked meats, you can eat to your heart's content. You must exclude beetroot salad, though, which contains sugar, and also carrots and sweetcorn.

As far as eggs are concerned, as you know, there is no restriction on their consumption, even if they come with mayonnaise[1]. Yes, mayonnaise, like crème fraîche, is permissible in a protein-lipid meal. That does not mean you should go overboard on it, but if you enjoy it, you can eat it in normal quantities. If you have a tendency to a high cholesterol level, though, it is better to avoid both mayonnaise and cream (see Chapter II and Chapter VIII).

As a starter, you can also have tuna, sardines in oil, crab, scampi or salmon, smoked or marinaded. In Phase I, though, it is better to avoid *oysters, scallops and foie gras,* all of which contain some carbohydrate and are likely to slow your progress, without actually sabotaging your plans completely. Do not worry; you will be able to eat them when you like in Phase II.

Main course

Essentially, your main dish will be fish or meat. There are no restrictions here, except in the way it is cooked, although eating more fish is desirable.

Meat and fish *must not be breadcrumbed.* Breadcrumbs are carbohydrate. Similarly, fish must not be

---

1. If you eat mayonnaise from a tube or jar, check its ingredients. There is a strong likelihood it contains sugar, glucose or some sort of flour.

coated in flour, so be wary of sole meunière. Always ask for your fish to be *grilled*.

Also to be avoided are gravies made from the pan juices, which are not always easily digested and, above all, are not good for the cholesterol level.

Beware of sauces! If you are a " nouvelle cuisine " enthusiast, you will find that sauces are usually light, insofar as they contain no flour. They are usually made from diluting the cooking juices and adding light crème fraîche.

If you eat meat, you can if you like have a sauce, such as a béarnaise[1], as long as you do not have cholesterol problems. But avoid too much mustard. In Phase I you can use just a teaspoonful in an oil and vinegar dressing, though, without doing any great harm.

To accompany your main course, your priority will be to choose whatever fibre-containing vegetables are available, ranging from tomatoes to courgettes, via French beans, aubergines, cauliflower — the choice is endless. Consult the list in the Appendix to get used to recognising the many vegetables on it[2].

As I have already said, if you are in a restaurant and none of these happens to be available, just choose a green salad : lettuce, lamb's lettuce, curly endive, or whatever. You can eat as much of this as you like, at whatever point in the meal you please.

---

1. Do not assume frozen vegetables are necessarily the exact equivalents of their fresh counterparts ; check packets to be sure they contain no added sugar.
2. Check the ingredients. In a restaurant it may well be made naturally with no sugar or other undesirable additives.

Cheese

From now on you must get used to eating cheese *without bread or biscuits.* It is not at all impossible and you will soon discover it actually tastes much better this way. And you will enjoy it all the more before long, when you are allowed to drink some wine with it.

In Phase I, more or less any kind of cheese is permitted. Exceptions need to be made for cantal and for goat cheeses, which contain a little carbohydrate, so it is better to avoid them in the early stages.

There is no reason why you should not finish a meal of this kind with a yogurt or some fromage frais, but do not eat more than 100 to 125g, because both do contain some carbohydrate. Anyone who is overweight and still very sensitive to carbohydrate may find that, although their glycaemic index is very low, fromage frais or yogurt can trigger an undesirable secretion of insulin at the end of the meal, and that could result in body fat being formed from the contents of the main course.

Desserts

Some desserts can be made with artificial sweeteners, if they do not require lengthy cooking. Egg custards or similar desserts are possibilities.

Drinks

We have already noted that in Phase I all alcoholic drinks, including wine, should be avoided. Drink water or tea, or herbal teas if you prefer. But avoid sparkling waters, as these can cause bloating and upset your digestion.

In any case, I suggest you drink very little water with your meals, as you risk diluting the gastric juices, thereby upsetting your digestive system. At least, if you must drink, do not start doing so until half-way through the meal. Do not drink as soon as you sit down to eat; this is a deplorable habit people have fallen into, which accounts for a good many of the metabolic problems they run into in digesting their food. *Drink between meals, instead* (at least a litre of water a day). And see that you do!

A reminder that, if you have to eat a large meal while you are in Phase I, you must abstain from the alcoholic apéritif. Try a tomato juice or a Perrier instead. If you really cannot get out of accepting something alcoholic (if, for example, your host has made a kir for everyone), then do so, but do not drink it. Moisten your lips with it from time to time, to be seen to be taking part in the general conviviality of the occasion, but do not swallow any. Sooner or later you can find a convenient moment to " abandon " your glass somewhere without anyone noticing. If you find it difficult to get rid of, you can always use a little ingenuity. Put it down within reach of someone who is knocking the stuff back; people like this can generally be relied on to pick up someone else's glass by mistake, especially if it is full. As a rule, there is at least one of these individuals at every gathering. If all else fails, there is always the flower-pot, the champagne bucket, the open window in summer or the basin in the cloakroom.

Advice if you have to attend a social function when you are in Phase 1 :

Accept the glass of champagne that is handed to you, and hold on to it for a while. Put it to your lips from time to time if you can bear to do that without drinking any. Then discreetly put it down somewhere.

Party food, though, can constitute a real headache. But it need not be an insoluble problem.

There is no question of eating sandwiches, however dainty they are. But what is in the sandwiches is good stuff : slices of salmon, sliced sausage, egg, asparagus, and so on. If you have the nerve and skill to separate the topping of an open sandwich from its base, good for you! Where there's a will, there's a way. But failing this, there is always party fare which comes within our rules.

Cherchez le fromage! There is always cheese around, in one form or another, in slices or, more usually, in little cubes.

Failing this, try to track down the cocktail sausages! But exercise restraint; think of the cholesterol!

If you think you are one of those people who just cannot resist a table laden with food, if you think you will inevitably succumb to temptation because when the hunger pangs strike your will-power will evaporate, then try this : before you go to the party, nibble something that is within the rules, to " line your stomach ".

In the mid-nineteenth century a forbear of mine (my great-great-grandfather), who had six children, was invited with his family to lunch with the managing director of the company he worked for. I am told that my great-great-grandmother took good care to see that the children were fed a hearty soup before they went. With their stomachs thus lined, these delightful children showed a good deal less unseemly enthusiasm than they might have done, when dishes of a magnificence they were quite unused to were set before them. And my great-great-grandparents acquired the instant reputation for having extremely well brought-up offspring.

So if you are afraid of giving in to temptation, eat a hard-boiled egg or a piece of cheese before you set off for your party. And you can get into the habit of always having with you some of those little individual cheeses like " Babybel " or " Laughing cow "[1].

These items can also be dipped into whenever you feel peckish, though dried fruit or high-fibre bread is even better. However, except for children, who should eat something at tea-time, hunger should not strike between meals, as long as your meals are well thought out and are high in fibre. In any case, do not confuse having tea and having a nibble between meals! And be careful about consuming lipids when you have had a carbohydrate meal. Do not, for

---

1. Again, this advice is for those who have no cholesterol problem. If you have high blood cholesterol, you would do better to choose something high-fibre, such as apples or kiwis.

example, eat a piece of gruyère at 9 o'clock in the morning if you only breakfasted at 8 o'clock.

What if you are invited to friends'? This can be a trickier situation, and you will have less room for manoeuvre.

Well, let us look at various possibilities. Maybe these are friends that you know well? They may even be relatives. In that case, you will be relaxed enough with them to " put your cards on the table ". Ask them in advance what is on the menu. You need not be afraid, even, to make a suggestion or two.

But let us suppose that you do not know your hosts very well. In this case you will have to play it by ear. If the occasion is a very special one, it will be a meal in line with the occasion, and I should be surprised if rice, pasta or potatoes figured as a major part of the menu.

If there is foie gras, go ahead and eat it, even though it is not to be recommended as food to be eaten freely in Phase I. But just once in a while it will do no harm. But please *do not eat the toast served with it.* There is no reason why you should; even politeness does not demand it.

If you are served a magnificent cheese soufflé, you can eat it along with everyone else, even though it will contain flour. But knowing that it puts you " in the red ", exercise restraint. Do not make a bad situation worse by accepting a third helping.

If the starter is a pâté en croûte, you can eat the pâté, which is generally protein-lipid, and leave the crust discreetly on the side of your plate. Given that you are not among close friends, no-one is likely to be rude enough to remark that you are " leaving the best part "! And even if the hostess is wondering why you did not like her pastry, she is unlikely to ask you outright.

When it comes to the main course, I should think you would have no difficulty, as the accompaniments are usually optional. You can take a symbolic helping of rice or pasta, but no-one can make you eat it.

If all this leaves you still starving, you can make up for it with the salad, if there is one, and, particularly, with the cheese. If you help yourself generously to the cheese, your hostess will be pleased and will find it easier to forgive you for leaving the crust from your pâté. An attractive cheese-board needs to have a good range of varieties, and guests rarely try many of them because they have no room after all the bread they have eaten. So it is up to you to do justice to the cheese-board!

The dessert is likely to be the most critical point of the meal, as it is always hard to say " no, thank you ". So insist on a *very small portion* and, like others who have eaten too much already, you can leave a substantial part of it on your plate.

Wait as long as possible into the meal before you start to drink. Give priority to drinking some red wine with the cheese.

Should the whole situation turn out to be worse than you expected, and, despite being still in Phase I, all your ingenuity could not protect you from the assaults of the bad carbohydrates, then your only recourse is to be more vigilant than ever thereafter in pursuit of your new way of eating.

You must realise that in Phase I you are still very sensitive to glucose. The object of this phase is to raise your tolerance level; as long as it has not reached a satisfactory level, *your sensitivity to glucose remains high.*

Obviously, if after denying your body bad carbohydrate for a while, you quite suddenly feed it a huge quantity, your metabolism will have a field day. And in a single evening you will bump up your fat reserves by more than the amount you have taken up to a fortnight to lose.

The further you are into Phase I (which should last at least two or three months), the less catastrophic the effect will be.

On the other hand, if you " go overboard " two or three weeks after starting Phase I, you run the risk of returning virtually to square one. This can be pretty discouraging. If this happens, you will just have to tell yourself that although you may have lost a battle, you still have a good chance of winning the war.

EVENING MEAL

This will be either protein-lipid with fibre or protein-carbohydrate with fibre.

Evening meal number 1

A protein-lipid and fibre evening meal will be just like a protein-lipid and fibre lunch. The only difference is that more often than not you will be eating at home. And at home, the choices are always more limited. But if you have been able to persuade your spouse and family to adopt your new eating habits too, you will have no difficulty. The ideal way to begin the meal is with a hearty thick vegetable soup. You can use turnips, leeks, celery, cabbage : any vegetables as long as they are listed in Appendix 1. Do not be tempted to pop in a potato, considered by many to be an essential ingredient. Of course, what the potato does is to thicken the soup, but this can also be done with celery, or by adding an egg yolk or some pureed mushrooms.

When serving your soup you can add a knob of butter or a little crème fraîche, unless, of course, you are watching your cholesterol level.

It is better to avoid meat in the evening, unless you eat poultry. Try eating eggs instead, and, above all, fish.

Avoid cooked meats and pâté in the evening, especially if you have eaten beef, veal, lamb or pork at midday, as the total saturated fats for the day could be putting your cholesterol level at risk.

When it comes to dairy products, cheese is permitted here too, but it is a good idea to alternate it with yogurt. These days we understand a good deal about the nutritive value of yogurt. It is known, for example, that it helps replenish the intestinal flora. It has recently been discovered that it also helps keep blood cholesterol down, boosts resistance to infection and helps keep constipation at bay. But be careful! Only eat good yogurt, without flavourings or fruit. And make sure that it is naturally fermented. You will not go wrong if you buy farmhouse yogurt or yogurt with bifidus[1].

---

1. Yogurt is nevertheless a carbohydrate-lipid combination, so you are not recommended to eat it at every meal.

Meals at home are the time to eat any of the simple, permitted foods that you enjoy. Pot-au-feu, for example, or mackerel, or sardines. Eat things which you are unlikely to find in a restaurant, like boiled artichokes, which are delicious, full of vitamins and minerals and rich in fibre to help intestinal function and bring down your blood glucose level. Above all, eat vegetables : tomatoes, spinach, chicory, aubergines, cauliflower, leeks, courgettes, mushrooms, ratatouille...

Evening meal number 2

This one is protein-carbohydrate and high in fibre. The carbohydrates will have a low glycaemic index and all forms of lipid will be excluded.

This meal can be made up from any of the following dishes :

— vegetable soup (without potato or carrots)
— wholegrain rice with a tomato and basil sauce or a purée of mushrooms and very low fat fromage frais
— haricot beans or red kidney beans
— artichoke with a vinaigrette of lemon, mustard and very low fat yogurt
— salad with a similar seasoning

and for dessert, good old " very low fat " fromage frais pepped up with a little fruit preserve.

It goes without saying that you will avoid all lipids : butter, oil, margarine, grated cheese, eggs, and so on.

You can eat this sort of meal two or three times a

week. It will help you to balance up your diet by using good carbohydrates, particularly pulses (lentils and beans) which contain vegetable protein.

You may also like to know that not eating fats in the evening is an additional aid to slimming. It is now known that it is the fats consumed at an evening meal that are most readily converted into body fat.

PICNICS

I expect that, for a variety of reasons, it often happens that you have no time to get a meal. Usually the mid-day meal is the one it is tempting to go without, the simplest thing being either to skip it completely or to make do with a quick sandwich.

Never, ever, skip a meal. This is one of the golden rules of nutrition. There is nothing to stop you eating four or five times a day, if you want to, but above all, do not miss out on one of the three main meals. It is the biggest mistake you can make, the quickest way to upset your whole metabolism. Do not allow yourself to do it, and discourage others from it too. If you miss meals, your body will behave like the dog which is not fed regularly; as soon as it is given anything to get its teeth into, it starts to store it away.

I am sure that by this stage you would not even consider the option of the ham sandwich from your favourite bar, or the infamous little burger bap. At the end of the book I will tell you exactly what I think of the appalling eating habits which have been exported to us from the country which is thought of as the pinnacle of Western civilisation. It is a land which certainly deserves our respect and admiration on a number of grounds, but definitely not on gastronomic or nutritional ones. So what are you going to eat instead of these horrors? Well, it just means combining what you now know with a little ingenuity.

Here are a few examples at random of some of the convenient things which will make an admirable snack at the work-place or keep you going when you are travelling :

— *Ham* [1] (smoked or unsmoked) : I particularly recommend Parma ham, because it is always sold in very thin slices which do not need a knife or fork.

— *Continental sausage* [1] : If you do not buy it ready-sliced, you may need a knife, but maybe your paper-knife will do.

— *Hard-boiled eggs* : readily found in delicatessens, bars and sandwich-shops.

— *Tomatoes* : ideal, as long as you take the precaution of having a supply of tissues to hand. Botanically the tomato is a fruit, but nutritionally it is considered a vegetable.

— *Cheese* : any kind will do, but as we need to be strictly *practical* in this section, we had better rule out brie, camembert and the like, whose friendly advances may be less than appreciated by those around you, especially on a train. There are plenty of other kinds of cheese to choose from.

If you have eaten nothing for some time, you can, as I have already suggested, make a picnic meal entirely of

---

1. Not advisable if you have high blood cholesterol. Try smoked salmon or crabsticks instead.

fruit. You can eat it to your heart's content, until you are full up. The only problem with fruit is that it is quite quickly digested, so a couple of hours later you may feel peckish again. You can always eat another apple or a piece of wholemeal bread. But even in an emergency, never resort to forbidden bad carbohydrates, like biscuits or, even worse, pseudo-chocolate covered snack bars and other such snacks.

If you practise a sport in the evening, you can eat some dried fruit a quarter of an hour or so beforehand.

The energy provided by the carbohydrate will be burned up immediately because your activity will involve using your muscles.

We have now dealt thoroughly with Phase I.

If, before adopting these new eating rules, you were used to eating sugar or were particularly fond of cakes and sweet things, you may lose 9 to 12 pounds in the first month. But do not stop there, or you risk putting all that weight back on again. Above all, you must avoid a pattern of expanding and contracting like an accordion.

After this first spell, the rate of weight loss will slow down, but continuing to follow the rules will result in your shedding weight gently and progressively.

The weight loss should proceed at an even pace, although, as we have already discussed, the actual rate will vary with the individual.

Experience shows that men tend to find it easier than women to obtain the desired results, though this is not always the case for men who are suffering from anxiety or who are on certain courses of medical treatment (some types of medication do increase the patient's tendency to put on weight). Women are much more prone to fluid retention (before a period, or as a reaction to stress or emotional problems), which can affect their weight in the short term (over one week, for example). But that does not mean that women cannot achieve results which are just as good over a slightly longer term. Quite the reverse...

It has been noted, though, that some women do have more difficulty than others in achieving these results.

Four possible causes have been identified :

1. Anxiety, which stimulates an abnormal level of insulin secretion.

2. Hormonal disturbances in adolescence or around the menopause.

3. Thyroid problems, though these are rare.

4. Sometimes a woman's body will put up a particular kind of resistance, at least initially, as a result of excessive and repeated low-calorie diets in the past. These may also have led to a larger accumulation of fat cells.

If you previously had problems with your cholesterol level, you will no longer need to be concerned. Once you learn how to manage your lipid consumption sensibly, you should, in a very short time, be rid of this particular worry.

Avoid fats — we eat too much fat — but, above all, avoid saturated fats, which raise your blood cholesterol level, and choose those fats which lower the amount of bad cholesterol and increase good cholesterol.

This approach has been definitively recognised by the world's specialists, and the scientific literature supporting it is impressive (see Chapter VIII on High Blood Cholesterol).

Although it is not likely, it is just possible that your doctor may not be in complete agreement with this new line, and feels it goes against what he was taught. In this domaine as in many others, it takes time for opinion to evolve, even in the light of irrefutable scientific evidence.

If you follow the rules of Phase I, it is not possible for you to fail to lose weight. If you do, or if success is abnormally slow in coming, then you are doing something wrong.

The thing to do then is to draw up an exhaustive list of everything you eat from waking to bedtime. With the help of this book, you should be able to work out what is amiss.

For example, you may be eating far too much normal yogurt or fromage frais (which contain both carbohydrates and lipids), or you may be regularly eating soups which you have been assured contain only " permitted " vegetables like tomatoes, sorrel and leeks. Be more suspicious and check out what the ingredients really are. You may discover, for example, that the soups come from tins or packets. If you read the information which is legally bound to be printed on the label, you may be amazed to find that, besides the permitted vegetables, there are also bad carbohydrates in the shape of starch, sugars, dextrose and other colourings or thickening agents.

So be vigilant! Even though the basic principles of the Method are easy enough to put into practice, they do necessitate, at least at first, some effort and, admittedly, some sacrifices. So do not risk doing all this for nothing by letting silly mistakes occur.

A word of warning. If you are currently on a low-calorie diet, do not swap suddenly to applying this Method. Your body is feeling the frustrations of the rationing imposed on it, and the sudden consumption of a much larger quantity of food might encourage it to lay down reserves. You could risk putting on 4 to 7 pounds before you begin to lose any. To avoid this unwanted weight gain, just start to apply the Method, but count the calories too for a few more days, putting your ration up by 100 calories a day.

DURATION OF PHASE I

The very reasonable question that you are sure to be asking on reaching the end of this section is :

How long do I have to stay in Phase I ?

At the risk of irritating you, I would answer : " How long is a piece of string ? ", because in fact it depends on a large number of factors.

You could say that Phase I should last long enough to enable you to shed all your unwanted weight, while realising that how long this will be will vary from one individual to another.

Or to put it another way, Phase I ends when you have attained your ideal weight. To calculate what this should be you have only to turn to Chapter XIII.

But perhaps instead of referring to it as your " ideal weight " we ought to call it your stabilised weight or the weight at which you feel good. This is a sort of threshold weight, at which the body decides of its own accord to stop and to slim no further, and it is a highly individual concept.

If you need to lose, say, one and a half to two and a half stones, Phase I could last from a few weeks to a few months.

If you only have to lose nine to twelve pounds, you may be tempted to cut it short as soon as you have attained that objective.

I must remind you, though, that the aim of Phase I, quite apart from shedding those unwanted pounds, is to give your pancreas a rest and to persuade it to raise its glucose tolerance level. This takes at least 2 months.

Consequently, if you are in too much of a hurry to be done with Phase I, even though you may have lost the pounds in question, you may not yet have given your pancreas long enough to become really healthy again.

Supposing you had no interest in losing weight, but were just following the method in order to recapture greater physical and intellectual vitality, you would be faced with the same problem. You would be well advised to prolong Phase I for as long as possible, to bring permanent benefit to all your digestive and metabolic functions.

In practice, the question of the duration of Phase I need hardly occur, because the change-over to Phase II is made very gradually, not from one day to the next.

And you will find that Phase I is not hard to live with, since it does not involve depriving yourself of much.

In fact, you will find you feel so good about it that you may have difficulty in dragging yourself out of Phase I at all.

108

TO SUMMARISE THE MAIN PRINCIPLES OF PHASE I :

Never mix bad carbohydrates (white bread, flour, starchy foods) *with lipids* (meat, fats, oils) *in the course of a meal.*

Avoid all carbohydrate-lipids (chocolate, avocado, liver, nuts, chips, pastries).

Eliminate sugar completely from your diet.

Eat only unrefined flours.

Eat only wholemeal bread, 100 % stoneground or with bran, made from unrefined flours (and then only for breakfast).

Forget about potatoes, especially chips.

Forget about white rice. Eat only (and in moderation) wholegrain or wild rice.

Never eat pasta made with refined flours. Eat wholewheat pasta.

Introduce pulses into your diet, especially as a main supper dish.

Temporarily give up all forms of alcohol, whether apéritif, wine, beer or digestif. This is essential in Phase I. Wine can be reintroduced later in reasonable amounts.

Avoid strong coffee. Get into the habit of drinking decaffeinated.

Never skip a meal. Spread your food intake over three meals, preferably always taken at the same times.

Restrict consumption of " bad" lipids, in favour of " good " lipids, with a view to warding off cardiovascular disease (see Chapter II).

Try to drink very little at meals to avoid diluting the gastric juices. Never drink immediately before you eat.

Take your time to eat. Chew food well and try to relax over meals.

Make your own fruit juices. Avoid commercially available fruit juices and soft drinks, which contain sugar.

Wait for three hours after a carbohydrate meal (breakfast, for example) *before consuming lipids.*

Wait for three to four hours after a lipid meal before consuming carbohydrates.

Eat plenty of dietary fibre : salads, pulses, green vegetables, fruit (see list in Chapter II).

Warning : The list above is only a summary of some of the principles discussed in the text. In no circumstances should it be taken as a condensed version of the method. Applying the method in a random way, without a full understanding of the preceding and following chapters, could result in nutritional imbalance and could be dangerous if the rules on consumption of lipids are not observed.

Note : As we have made the first part of this journey, we have become acquainted with two kinds of carbohydrate, the " good " sort which can be consumed without fear of putting on weight, and the " bad " sort, which must be systematically tracked down and eliminated. The difference between them lies not only in the proportion of carbohydrate in a particular food but, more importantly, the way in which it releases glucose during the digestive process. The more refined a flour, the more it has to be considered a

" bad " carbohydrate. The nearer bread comes to being 100 % stoneground wholemeal, made from unprocessed cereal high in dietary fibre, the more it qualifies as a " good " carbohydrate (see Chapter II).

Examples of PHASE I menus

Midday meals :

Tomato salad	Cucumber salad
Rabbit with parsley	Fillet of cod in tomato sauce
French beans	Spinach
Cheese	Yogurt
To drink : water or weak or herbal tea	To drink : water or weak or herbal tea
Radishes with butter	Mackerel in white wine
Turkey escalope	Grilled beefburger
Braised chicory	Broccoli
Cheese	Yogurt
To drink : water or weak or herbal tea	To drink : water or weak or herbal tea
Mushroom salad	Hearts of palm
Roast chicken	Pork chop
Courgette gratin	Pureed celery
Cheese	Yogurt
To drink : water or weak or herbal tea	To drink : water or weak or herbal tea
Leeks in vinaigrette	Celeriac with oil and mustard dressing
Grilled kidneys	Leg of lamb
Salsifi	Courgette gratin
Cheese	Yogurt
To drink : water or weak or herbal tea	To drink : water or weak or herbal tea
Sardines in oil	Asparagus
Frankfurters	Black pudding
Cabbage	Cauliflower purée
Cheese	Yogurt
To drink : water or weak or herbal tea	To drink : water or weak or herbal tea

Endive salad with bacon pieces Grilled chicken Peas Cheese To drink : water or weak or herbal tea	Meat consommé Pot-au-feu Turnips, leeks, cabbage Yogurt To drink : water or weak or herbal tea
Smoked salmon Duck breast Mushrooms with parsley Green salad, cheese To drink : water or weak or herbal tea	Tuna in oil Steak tartare Green salad Yogurt To drink : water or weak or herbal tea
Red cabbage Skate with capers Pureed French beans Cheese To drink : water or weak or herbal tea	Smoked ham Grilled salmon Spinach Yogurt To drink : water or weak or herbal tea
Mozzarella cheese Veal escalope Brussels sprouts Cheese To drink : water or weak or herbal tea	Eggs mimosa Entrecôte Aubergines Yogurt To drink : water or weak or herbal tea

Note : If you have a high cholesterol level, most cheeses must be ruled out ; you can eat a green salad instead or choose a low-fat cheese.
Note : Avoid cheese alternately mid-day and evening, alternating with yogurt.

Evening meals — protein-lipid with fibre

Home-made vegetable soup	Fish soup
Fried eggs	Unsmoked ham
Ratatouille	Green salad
1 full-fat yogurt	Cheese
To drink : water or herbal tea	To drink : water or herbal tea
Vegetable soup	Artichokes with vinaigrette
Stuffed tomatoes (see Appendix IV for recipe)	Scrambled egg with tomatoes
Green salad	Green salad
1 full-fat yogurt	
To drink : water or herbal tea	To drink : water or herbal tea
Onion soup	Vegetable soup
Tuna flan (see Appendix IV for recipe)	Cold chicken breasts in mayonnaise
Green salad	Green salad
Strained fromage frais	Cheese
To drink : water or herbal tea	To drink : water or herbal tea
Mozzarella, tomato and basil salad	Mushroom salad
Aubergine gratin (see Appendix IV for recipe)	Stuffed aubergines
Chicory salad	Green salad
	Strained fromage frais
To drink : water or herbal tea	To drink : water or herbal tea
Cucumber in low-fat « cream »	Asparagus
Sorrel omelette	Poached fillet of white fish
Green salad	Spinach
	Cheese
To drink : water or herbal tea	To drink : water or herbal tea

114

Evening meals — protein-carbohydrate with fibre

Vegetable soup (home-made) Wholegrain or wild rice in tomato 1 « very low fat » yogurt	Vegetable soup (home-made) Wholewheat pasta in tomato Strained « very low fat » fromage frais
Lentils (« very low fat » fromage frais cheese sauce) Salad with lemon juice 1 « very low fat » yogurt	Baked tomatoes with parsley Dried beans (« very low fat » fromage frais cheese sauce) 1 « very low fat » yogurt
Vegetable curry (avoiding recipes with fats, « very low fat » yogourt can be used) Wholegrain rice	Cucumber in fat-free cream dressing Aubergines stuffed with mushroom purée and « very low fat » fromage frais 1 « very low fat » yogurt

Note : It is crucial not to consume any fat in the course of these carbohydrate meals.

PHASE II : MAINTAINING
A STABLE WEIGHT

So here we are approaching " cruising speed " and you have a complete understanding of the principles underlying your new way of eating. You have out-lawed permanently certain " dangerous " foods, and for some weeks now you have been refining your new eating habits. As a result, you have reached your goal of losing however many pounds you needed to and now you are ready to go on to Phase II.

Unlike Phase I, which by definition was to last for a limited period, Phase II will undoubtedly be with you for the rest of your life. Personally, I have been in Phase II for getting on for ten years, and I have not put on an ounce. And yet I never deprive myself of anything.

Phase II, as the section heading indicates, is about *maintaining a stable weight*. This is the stage at which we are really going to learn to manage our eating.

In Phase I, we mainly cut out certain foodstuffs, and at times I spoke sternly of items being forbidden. In Phase II nothing, or hardly anything, is completely forbidden. There will just be a few things to avoid, and then only under specific conditions.

So in Phase II the guiding principles will seem less rigid, more open to interpretation. In other words, the real art of management comes in.

And management is not just a matter of blindly following a set of rules which have been meticulously laid down for all time. It is also to do with interpret-ing rules appropriately. Any idiot can follow rules rigidly, as we know only too well from all those bureaucracies, public and private, which believe in the regulations, the whole regulations and nothing but the regulations. I am not now asking you to " administer " your diet, as you did in Phase I, because, from now on, this would be boring and unnecessary. Management (in the true sense of the word) has the subtlety of an art, which mere administration has not. The " third clerk on the left " simply follows the rules ; the good manager draws inspiration from them.

So this is rather what I am suggesting to you here.

We will take another look at the basic rules, but stopping along the way to see how we can now interpret and apply them creatively.

Sugar

This remains, and always will remain, a dangerous product. What I said in Phase I still holds true here. Get into the habit of excluding it from your diet. Even if you do not have your sweetener with you, do not give in to the temptation to say to yourself : " Just one little lump of sugar wouldn't really be a disaster. " True though that might be in one sense, it is only valid reasoning if you can be absolutely certain that you have not consumed and will not consume another single bad carbohydrate all day.

So stand firm! No sugar lumps in your coffee! No sugar sprinkled on your fromage frais! Either use your sweetener, or do without!

The basis of Phase II is that from now on you can take considerable liberties compared to Phase I. But do not take your freedom for granted ; you must consider yourself *on probation.* Your freedom is conditional and you must manage your behaviour accordingly!

You will, in fact, find yourself " forced " to eat sugar, because it is present in most desserts. I will show you how to choose the ones which have least. But if you decide to give in to your yearning to eat a dessert, then you cannot also put a lump of sugar in your coffee. Drink your coffee unsweetened if you can, but never give in to the temptation of putting sugar in it.

I repeat, *stand firm* against sugar! It is a poison and should be treated as such!

You will find that you can be more self-indulgent with other items.

And what about honey? This is a question you have probably been dying to ask from the start. As it is a natural, unrefined product, you are probably expecting me to be all in favour.

I am afraid I have to disappoint you somewhat. What we have to be concerned with in honey is the glycaemic index of the carbohydrate.

Unfortunately, it has a high glycaemic index of 90, and therefore has to count as a bad carbohydrate.

It has few nutritional virtues. On the other hand, if you are consuming it for its medicinal properties, you can, if you must, take a teaspoonful a day for the few days' duration of the course of treatment. It can be taken, for example, at the end of a carbohydrate breakfast.

Bread

One of my brothers is, like me, a great enthusiast for good red wines. The full consequences of eating bread at a main meal really came home to him when I told him : " Every time you eat one mouthful of bread, you will have to abstain from one glass of Bordeaux-". Everything is a matter of choice !

At breakfast, if you are eating a carbohydrate meal, you must go on eating *only stoneground or other wholemeal bread* (see Chapter V, Breakfast). If after three months, though, you have " very low fat " from-age frais " coming out of your ears ", you can now replace it with margarine or a low-fat spread contain-ing butter, as long as you only use a small amoun-t. Eat butter only very rarely and if you really have no choice — when you are away from home, for example.

The same goes for milk. On principle, stick to the habit of consuming only skimmed milk. If, on occa-sion, you have none to hand, as can happen if you are away from home, use semi-skimmed.

The carbohydrate breakfast recommended in Phase I leaves plenty of room for manoeuvre, so organise yourself so as to stick to it permanently.

From time to time, I have to attend working break-fasts at big Paris hotels. On these occasions I usually cannot resist trying the delicious brioches or the wonderful croissants oozing with butter.

At the end of breakfast, though, I automatically make a mental note of this *discrepancy* on my dietary balance-sheet. By this I mean that I shall keep it in mind when I come to choose what to eat at lunch and dinner. Probably, I shall refrain from eating a chocolate dessert at lunch, or I shall abstain from wine, if possible, at dinner.

By now you will have got the basic idea of what good management of your diet involves : *distributing the discrepancies evenly.* The body has a certain level of tolerance to a mixture of lipids and good carbohydrates. And as long as you do not go beyond this reasonable limit, you will be able to maintain your ideal weight.

I cannot tell you exactly where this limit lies, for it varies with individuals, depending on their sensitivity to glucose and the way in which their pancreas reacts. If you have taken Phase I seriously and raised your glucose tolerance threshold, it is probable that insulin production will now be under much better control and it will be present only in those quantities needed to remove excess glucose from your bloodstream. But, do not worry, you will very easily discover for yourself where this threshold lies, just by weighing yourself regularly.

It goes without saying that a good manager will keep a permanent eye on the warning lights, and you will monitor your weight just as you monitor your personal budget. You will know that discrepancies are always easy to correct if you spot them in time.

At lunch, whether at home, at work or in a restaurant, stick to another of the golden rules : *no white bread with your meal!* If you are eating oysters, it is preferable to eat three or four more of them, carbohydrate-lipid mixture though they are, than to eat a piece of white bread with butter.

120

If you eat smoked salmon in a restaurant, do not eat the toast served with it. Or you could order fresh marinaded salmon instead : delicious, and it will not be served with toast, so temptation will not be put in your way.

If you eat foie gras, the toast is again a no-go area, especially given that the liver is something of a carbohydrate-lipid. This is one reason why it was not in the list of permitted foods in Phase I.

By doing without bread except at breakfast, you will gradually find you are savouring more fully the dishes you are served. This is particularly true of foie gras, a delicacy I would always encourage you to choose in a restaurant where it is fresh. You can always eat the preserved sort at home. There is another rule for you (Not that it is anything to do with the object of this book ; it is more one of the basis rules of gastronomy) : *in a restaurant, eat the things you cannot eat at home.*

When I am in a restaurant I am often amazed at the conservatism of those I am with, be they French people or foreigners. They look at the menu, and invariably settle for classic dishes or whatever is most run-of-the-mill ; in other words, they eat what they can eat any day of the week, whether they are at home or abroad. It can take all the maître d'hôtel's powers of diplomacy and persuasion to deflect them from the commonplace dish which most resembles what they usually eat.

If they are as unimaginative and unadventurous in their work, I pity their bosses, shareholders or colleagues.

If you happen to be in France, fish is a wise choice in a restaurant. Most of the great French cooks demonstrate the very best of their talent when creating fish dishes. France is one of the few countries in the world where, even 500km from the coast, you can always find good fresh fish. So make the most of it and encourage this happy state of affairs.

Coming back to bread... I will allow you one small concession when it comes to the cheese course. If you are in France and in one of the few places where they serve wholemeal bread, and provided you have not yet introduced into your meal any discrepancy of note, I would not wish to deprive you of the particular pleasure of the combination of chèvre cendré (goat's cheese ripened in ashes), wholemeal bread and a glass of maturing Médoc.

Starchy foods

Even in Phase II, I retain my healthy distrust of potatoes, white rice, white pasta and corn.

In Phase I, you will have learnt that these, together with white bread, are the major culprits when it comes to weight gain, and that whenever they are mixed with lipids, their effects are catastrophic. So, like bread, it is better to do without them, both at lunchtime and in the evening, unless you deliberately decide to make an exception.

There is, though, a way of minimising the negative effects of these bad carbohydrates. By eating fibre with them, you can in fact reduce their glycaemic index.

For example, if you decide to indulge in the sheer pleasure of eating chips, be sure to accompany them with a generous helping of salad. The fibre will reduce the seriousness of the discrepancy which the chips will certainly represent. You will sometimes find yourself in situations where a discrepancy is impossible to avoid. But do not just give in as a matter of course. What I am trying to say is that you should " *condition* " yourself to reject instinctively any such discrepancy, without giving it a second thought. Even if you manage to do this, the occasions when you are forced to make exceptions to the rules will be numerous enough to satisfy any flights of fancy you may have.

In " nouvelle cuisine " restaurants, where everything is served on your plate, there are usually three or four accompanying vegetables, and no-one will hold it against you if you leave one.

But then again, you may be invited to your neighbour's or to your crotchety old aunt's. And if you leave the smallest mouthful of potato or the least grain of rice stuck to your plate, your family relationships may be in tatters. In that case, you will just have to resign yourself to an extra discrepancy, frustrating though it may be if it has occasioned you no compensatory pleasure.

Remember, though, that whether or not you actually enjoyed finishing up your bad carbohydrates, you will have to cancel them out, either by forgoing the wine, or by declining the dessert. If you are unfortunate enough not only to have to eat up your rice, but also to have to demolish the stodgy baba au rhum which your hostess has gone to the trouble of making for you, you will be seriously " into the red ". Depending on the extent of your discrepancies, you may even need to go back to Phase I for a day or two to balance things up.

However, even in such desperate instances, fight against the temptation to think that the battle is lost and that you may as well go back to your old ways. And the urge to tell yourself, as you give in, that you can always decide on what action to take when you see the extent of the damage. This is *an ever-present danger, which you must resist at all costs.*

And never let slip your observance of the rules on the pretext that " they are impossible to stick to over Christmas, anyway ".

A numbers of years' experience has taught me that, however critical the situation, managing your eating habits always remains possible. If you are forced to introduce discrepancies, so be it, but just remember to compensate, then and later, by at least avoiding what can be avoided. If you start applying the principles of the Method on a " roller-coaster " basis, you will never get anywhere with it.

What it is all about, as you now know, is raising your glucose tolerance level as much as possible. If you decide you can always go back to Phase I when you put on half a stone, you really will not succeed in doing this.

I can tell you from my own experience that, after ten years of good Phase II management, my glucose tolerance threshold is very high. This shows that the more careful you are in the early years, the more you can subsequently accommodate large discrepancies.

The Method I am suggesting *to you aims to break you of the bad habits you have been acquiring* since childhood. One of the keys to success lies in "*positive reconditioning*". If this is done successfully in Phase I, you will find Phase II practically effortless. You

124

will have acquired a number of automatic reactions which will permanently ensure that you make the right decisions in managing your diet.

So if you see fresh pasta on a menu and are tempted to order it, go ahead, but do so knowing what you are doing. Savour the pleasure to the full, but make a mental note to take action later to counter the negative effects.

Or let us suppose you have decided, in the course of one meal, to eat foie gras, oysters and scallops, without depriving yourself of the glass of Beaujolais which goes down so well with shellfish. If then in the depths of your main dish you discover a potato lurking, or some rice, or pasta, *avoid it like the plague!* You are not so weak, for goodness' sake, that you need to give in.

You are probably not convinced simply from reading all this that you will be capable of resisting or will have the will-power to leave on your plate some item you like.

Well, you will find that it is, in fact, much easier than you think. After your delight at the spectacular results you have achieved in Phase I, you will automatically hold back, and will actually find it quite hard to give in to these temptations.

And, little by little, you will discover that the situation becomes self-regulating and you will find yourself on automatic pilot, as it were.

Fruit

As far as fruit is concerned, these same rules apply here as in Phase I. You must always eat fruit on any empty stomach.

You will have gathered that what is behind this rule is not so much the relative quantity of carbohydrate (fructose or glucose) contained in the fruit as the fact that fruit eaten with anything else *is not properly digested.* If you read the relevant part of the book carefully, you will understand why this is. There are some fruits, though, which are so low in carbohydrates that there is no problem about eating them, every day if you want to, in Phase II. These are *strawberries, raspberries and blackberries.*

So, whether at lunch or dinner, at home or in a restaurant, eat strawberries and raspberries.

If your meal is strictly protein-lipid, you can even add a little light crème fraîche. But be careful not to put sugar on your fruit; use a sweetener if you feel the need.

If you have indulged in no discrepancies (except wine), or if your discrepancies have been very minor ones, you can even have crème Chantilly (whipped cream), even though a small amount of sugar may have been added. At home, of course, you can make your " Chantilly " with a sweetener.

Another fruit you can eat with no problems in Phase II is melon — at the start of the meal, of course. If you do eat it as a starter, try and wait just a quarter of an hour, if you can, before going on to the next course, especially if it is fish or meat, as will usually be the case in a restaurant. If melon is served as a component of the hors-d'oeuvre, you can quite happily eat it mixed with any other salads, except those containing eggs, mayonnaise or cooked meats. But, there again, this advice is given with digestive problems in mind.   The risk of putting on weight in Phase II from eating melon is extremely small.

A number of readers of previous editions of this book wrote in to ask whether cooked fruit should be treated in the same way as raw fruit.   I am inclined to say it should, but with a few subtle exceptions.   Cooked fruit will ferment less than raw fruit, so that there is less gastric disturbance.   So a helping of stewed fruit, a pear Hélène or a peach melba will only constitute a very small discrepancy.

You must realise, on the other hand, that the fibre in cooked fruit has lost the major part of its value, particularly its property of reducing blood sugar. Cooked fruit also contains less vitamin C.

As for fruit in syrup, this should be ruled out completely, because of its high sugar concentration.

Dried fruits have a medium glycaemic index but most contain good fibre.   Dried figs, dried apricots or prunes can be consumed at times of high energy expenditure.

Desserts

This section, like the one on wine, is close to my heart, as I have by nature a sweet tooth — at any time, but particularly at the end of a meal.

We all have our weaknesses.   We just have to know how to control them.

Personally, I could do without potatoes for ever, and fresh pasta for at least a year, but I could never survive for more than a week without chocolate.

Within the " nouvelle cuisine " tradition there is also

" nouvelle pâtisserie ", and it has to be said that over the past ten years the great chefs — who are all great pâtissiers too — have come on by leaps and bounds in this field in terms of creativity and ingenuity.

French pâtisserie is far and away the best in the world, for its sheer originality, beauty, natural flavours and, in particular, its lightness.

In Phase II such delicacies will become available to you to enjoy, without any need for you to transgress our rules. If you like pastries, eat the lightest kinds, which also happen to be the best. Those which fit in best with our way of eating are naturally those which contain least flour and sugar. Just as " nouvelle cuisine " sauces contain no flour, so " nouvelle pâtisserie ", especially the mousses, contain little or no flour and always very little sugar. The recipe for bitter chocolate fondant in Appendix 3 contains only about 5 % flour, 50g in a cake weighing 1kg. And as for sugar, you do not need to add any at all. The small quantity contained in the dark chocolate you are using is quite enough. So here is one cake you can revel in while only notching up a small discrepancy on your daily balance sheet.

I can also recommend to you the chocolate mousse, which contains hardly any carbohydrate apart from the small quantity present in the dark chocolate. If it is not sweet enough for your taste (which would surprise me), simply add a little sweetener in powder form (see recipe in Appendix 3).

I began this section with chocolate, because it is a passion of mine. Partly because I love chocolate, and partly because, if it is top quality (which means it has

128

high cocoa content), it is low in carbohydrate and has a low glycaemic index of 221 [1].

But there are plenty of other things, just as delicious, among the " nouveaux desserts ". The bavarois, for example. This is a fruit mousse (choose strawberry or raspberry if you can) with a set consistency. It does contain sugar, and a few bad carbohydrates, but only in very modest quantity. Without going into the boring percentages, let us just say that your slice of bavarois contains less bad carbohydrate than a forkful of chips, a piece of toast or two or three biscuits.

Besides the bavarois, there is the charlotte, which I would describe as a sort of bavarois coated in biscuit. Enjoy the inner part, which is often frozen, and leave the biscuit, which is of no gastronomic interest and contains a high concentration of bad carbohydrate.

If you like ices, you do not need to deprive yourself of them, as their glycaemic index is only 35. The amount of sugar in good quality ice-cream is relatively low. Sorbets, however, have a glycaemic index of 65.

But if you have heard that because ice-cream is cold it is easily digested, do not believe it. It is only the momentary impression that it gives.

Maybe if you like ice-cream, you like it even more served with hot chocolate sauce and a mountain of whipped cream, delicately topped with a little Japanese umbrella. Well, you have no need to deprive yourself of this. As discrepancies go, it is not even equivalent to a modest helping of potatoes.

As for tarts and flans, of whatever type, they should

---

1. *Les vertus thérapeutiques du chocolat,* by Dr. Hervé Robert, published by Editions Artulen.

make you stop and think, because of the quantity of bad carbohydrate in the flour and sugar. But again, it is all a matter of choice. Your slice of flan is no worse than a baked potato or two tablespoons of white rice.

If you have had a day with no, or few, discrepancies, the choice is yours. But, as always, decide to eat a thing only if you will enjoy it and if you are sure that its quality will be worth the little sacrifice that will have to be made to balance things up again.

Alcohol

All alcoholic drinks should be subject to the same kind of management as food. In Phase II, as I explained to you, you will be able to reintroduce alcoholic drinks, but within certain limits. What I mean is that, here too, you will have to make choices. I warn you here and now that you will not be able to reintroduce in one fell swoop an apéritif, white wine, red wine and an after-dinner liqueur — if, indeed, this was what you used to consume. Even at a special meal (which will, by its very nature, involve you in other discrepancies too), it is just not on. You will have to manage your drinking in the same way that you manage your eating.

The apéritif

As an apéritif, it is better to drink a glass of wine or good champagne than spirits, such as whiskey, even if you add water or Perrier[1]. The discrepancy is simply

---

1. Tonic, on its own or with alcohol, is a sugared drink. Give it up!

smaller. One whiskey has as much alcohol as half a bottle of red wine. Personally, I would rather save up my discrepancy for the wine. That is why I never drink an apéritif in a restaurant, and very rarely at home. At apéritif time, and so as not to seem unsociable, I prefer to order a glass of wine. Generally I just ask the wine waiter to bring us right away the wine we are going to drink with the meal. A young Bordeaux or a Beaujolais supérieur goes with almost anything, so that you do not need to have decided on the complete order before you choose your wine. Anyway, you can always order another wine during the course of the meal, even just a half-bottle, if need be.

I am sure it is unnecessary to urge you not to drink more than one apéritif, especially if it is something like whiskey. In the improbable event that you really cannot avoid it, then make sure you are drinking wine or champagne.

Apéritif time is generally the hardest part when you are managing your eating carefully. If you are at friends' it can drag on for ages, as the hostess will often wait until everyone has arrived before she puts the final touches to the meal, and this in itself can take the best part of an hour.

If you politely arrived on time, you can find yourself faced with a two-hour apéritif. This can seem a long time if there are only bad carbohydrates to nibble away at, and if you have decided to save your discrepancies for the excellent red wines your host has laid down in his cellar or the delicious raspberry dessert that your hostess specialises in.

The occasions which I find particularly nightmarish are parties in English-speaking countries, where you may be invited for as early as half past six, even if you arrive an hour later, and you may have to last out until nine or ten o'clock before food is served.

I have unhappy memories of one evening at the home of an English family who had just come to live in the outskirts of Paris. At midnight one French couple got up to leave and were amazed when their hostess said, in her charming English accent, " Oh, you're not going, are you? We're just going to eat." The couple had arrived very punctually at seven o'clock, imagining that the English must eat very early. Four hours later, after refusing any drinks beyond the first one, and in a full-blown state of hypoglycaemia, they were getting quite desperate.

If you have experienced this kind of party, you have no doubt been amazed at the quantity of alcohol people seem able to consume on an empty stomach. You may also have noticed how the main preoccupation of your host on these occasions is to keep topping up his guests' glasses. One problem is that you cannot keep track of how much you are drinking, but this seems to be the least of people's worries. Another habit in English-speaking countries is that of taking an unfinished apéritif with you when you are asked to move to the dining-table. Maybe there is some logic in this, since if your host has been " topping you up ", you will inevitably have a full glass when the moment arrives.

I have said a good deal about apéritif time, but only to point out that it can represent a *snare* and needs careful management. But in my experience you can always get round the problems if you really want to.

In any case, remember that the first rule is to eat

something protein-lipid beforehand (cheese, cooked meats, fish), because drinking on an empty stomach is not only sacrilege, it is above all the start of a metabolic disaster.

Wine

I have several times mentioned the subject of wine and you will have gathered that my own preferences are directed towards red wine in general and Bordeaux in particular.

You are correct in your deduction, and I will explain why. This does not mean, though, that I reject white wines or red wines other than Bordeaux. Once again, it is a matter of choice within your food management programme.

I concede, for example, that the best wine to go with a really good foie gras is a Sauternes, especially if you are lucky enough to have in front of you an outstandingly good, fresh foie gras. But *management is the art of compromise!*

Liver, as you know, is a carbohydrate-lipid, which means that it constitutes a discrepancy, however small. Sauternes being a sweet wine, constitutes another. If you play all your *wild cards* at the start of the meal, how are your management techniques going to deal with the rest of it?

But it is up to you to decide whether to drink the Sauternes, as long as you keep it to a strict minimum, just the amount you need to enjoy your foie gras. Just keep in mind that a glass of Sauternes is about equivalent to three glasses of Médoc.

Given that at a normal meal we can drink several glasses of wine without upsetting our carbohydrate-lipid balance, we may as well drink a wine with less sugar in it, which will be a smaller discrepancy. In general, this is the advantage of red wines and dry white wines.

But while recommending red wines, there are nevertheless some important distinctions to be drawn. In the hierarchy of suitability I would give top place to young red wines with an alcohol content of between 9 and 12 degrees. In this category you will find Beaujolais, Gamay, Loire wines like Chinon, Bourgueil, Anjou, Saumur, Champigny and a number of other little vins de pays which are drunk young, such as wines from Savoie. Of course, the further south you go, the higher the alcohol content of the wines. But that is no reason to rule them out.

I think that in Phase II it is possible to have three glasses of red wine without putting at risk the general balance of our new way of eating. As an example, take the following, perfectly balanced meal :

Mushrooms à la grecque
Grilled sole with ratatouille
Green salad
Raspberries
Decaffeinated coffee

Drinking three glasses of wine with this meal will make you put on absolutely no weight, as long as you only start drinking towards the end of the main course, after you have already consumed enough food to neutralise, as it were, the effect of the alcohol. And, contrary to what you may fear, the wine will not have the side effect of sending you to sleep during the afternoon.

134

If you have to attend a meeting after lunch, you can observe that it is the people who have eaten bad carbohydrates, especially white bread, who will have a marked tendency to drop off. Paradoxically, they may have drunk nothing but water.

It is quite obvious that it would be even better if you drank no wine at all. But one of the aims of this book is to show you that, as long as you observe a few rules, you can continue both to meet your social and professional obligations and to satisfy your own tastes. On the other hand, if you are eating at home in the evening, drink water. It is not advisable to drink more than half a bottle of wine a day.

I have already pointed out that it seemed to me an important rule that you should not drink alcohol on an empty stomach. This is a principle I advise you to stick to.

Alcohol which is ingested on an empty stomach is absorbed immediately into the bloodstream, triggering the familiar metabolic process : the secretion of insulin and the laying down of fat reserves. It can also make you feel light-headed if you have not much experience of alcohol.

If, however, alcohol mingles with other foods in the stomach, the two will react with each other so that the alcohol is metabolised more slowly. The more slowly this happens, the less it will trigger off the undesirable side effects we have mentioned.

It is obvious therefore that the sensible advice is *to begin drinking as late as possible — even if you make up for it later in the meal.*

I would also advise you never to drink water with a

meal. This may appear contradictory, but let me explain my reasoning.

You have seen that, when you drink wine on a full stomach, it is metabolised more slowly, because the alcohol is first absorbed by other foods, and will be digested along with them. If these other foods are proteins or lipids (meat or fish, for example) which are, by definition, digested very slowly, the alcohol will also be metabolised that much more slowly. The slower the process, the less " fattening " the wine will be.

If you alternate drinking water and wine, you will simply dilute the wine with the water. This mixture will swamp the other foods rather than combine with them, will be metabolised quickly and will pass into your bloodstream as if you had drunk it on an empty stomach.

People will advise you to drink a lot of water to help eliminate organic waste products. This is fair enough, but drinking water at table, except in very modest quantities, is sacrilege. Firstly, it is bad for your digestion, as it dilutes the gastric juices too much, and secondly, it is the quickest way to metabolise any alcohol you may have drunk.

So get into the habit of drinking very little with your meals and, above all, do not drink water if you are drinking wine.

After-dinner drinks

Since discovering that wine is better metabolised if consumed late in the meal, you might expect me to advise you that a liqueur at the end your meal would do no more harm than a glass of Vichy water. I am afraid I am about to disappoint you.

The " little nip " to round off the meal can indeed be an aid to digestion ; that is why in France it is called a " digestif ". Alcohol has the property of dissolving fats, so if your meal was very rich in lipids, the alcohol may well help the digestive process.

My grandmother (a native of the Bordeaux region) passed away peacefully at the age of 102. Within living memory, she had never been known to finish a meal without a glass of a certain famous liqueur. And at table she had never drunk anything but Bordeaux. Certainly, I never saw her drink a glass of water at a meal.

My other grandmother (who came from the Gers, in the Armagnac region) died much younger, at the age of 99. She too enjoyed her little tot after a meal, but not necessarily after every meal.

Far be it from me to stick my neck out and deduce that they had both found the secret of longevity in their little " dram ". But you have to admit it makes you think.

Technically, I would say that if the meal has only been " washed down " in a very modest way, a drop of alcohol at the end can have no disastrous effects, especially if it really is only a drop.

On the other hand, if you decide to drink a cognac big enough to float a battleship, when you have already had four or five glasses of wine during the meal, I would not like to answer for the effect. One good glassful is about equivalent to three or four glasses of wine. Just do the arithmetic and " Disaster, here we come ! "

I leave it to you to draw your own conclusions.

Coffee

In Phase II, I would advise you to stick to the good habits you acquired in Phase I and drink only decaffeinated coffee. Since you will by now have overcome the tendency to " run out of steam " through hypoglycaemia or post-prandial torpor, the need for caffeine will have entirely disappeared. Giving up caffeine will do as much for you as giving up nicotine.

However, given that you will have considerably raised your tolerance threshold, at which insulin secretion is triggered, the possible ingestion of a small quantity of caffeine should not constitute a serious threat to your new-found dietary balance.

Other drinks

As far as other drinks are concerned, lemonades, fizzy drinks, milk and fruit juices, there is nothing much to add to what I said in Phase I. In Phase II just stick with the recommendations you were given before.

Conclusion

Phase II is both easier and harder to stick to. It is easier than Phase I in that it contains very few restrictions and even fewer forbidden foods. On the other hand, it is harder in that it demands skilled and subtle management, which must be strictly and permanently adhered to. So be vigilant and always on the look-out for ways of avoiding the pitfalls.

The first of these potential pitfalls is *management error*. Management error consists of only taking account of one factor at a time in managing your eating. For example : you drink a whiskey before your meal, but you then dutifully wait until you reach the main course to start on the three glasses of wine you are allowing yourself. Although you have correctly remembered that alcohol has less effect on a full stomach, do not expect spectacular results from your later behaviour when you have previously drunk your apéritif on an empty stomach.

At the end of this chapter, you will find a list of the golden rules for Phase II. Learn them by heart, so that you can apply them in a balanced way.

But the biggest pitfall is that of managing your eating like a yo-yo, alternating letting things slide completely with rushing back to a strict Phase I to salvage what you can. If you let yourself slip into following this kind of " method ", I give you three months before you are back to square one with those surplus pounds.

The goal you must set yourself — and this is the whole aim of the Method — is to achieve stability. And you will only do this by developing good management techniques for Phase II, which is for life. Even if you find Phase II a bit restrictive at first, it will get easier by the day. The more you practise the Method, the more managing your diet will become second nature, determined by habit and automatic reactions. In a word, you will have reconditioned yourself.

Do not let yourself be influenced or discouraged by those around you.

Equally, do not go to great lengths to win over people who have no desire to change their own eating habits. I made this mistake at the beginning, and tried to convert everyone to my new " religion ". But you should just mind your own business : manage your diet without feeling you have to tell your table companions about it. Even if the blatant errors they are making before your eyes do whip up your missionary zeal and give you a burning desire to rescue them from their own folly, do not try to help if they do not want to be helped. By trying to interfere, you will only make them feel aggressive or guilty. A good many of them know they are not eating sensibly, but they also know they do not have the willpower to break out of their bad habits.

As I have pointed out, Phase II gives you great freedom of choice, but you are " *on probation* ", as it were : your freedom has conditions attached.

Keep a permanent watch on your diet. Do not be a slave to your weight, but stay alert to it by monitoring it closely. Your scales should be sufficiently sensitive to give you an accurate view of the results of your discrepancies. Keep your ideal weight firmly in mind, and by trial and error you will learn how to keep it stable. If you are unfortunate enough to find yourself drifting away from it, do not change direction completely. Simply make the necessary adjustment to get back on course. You will find that little by little you will go over to " automatic pilot " without even realising it is happening.

140

SUMMARY OF PHASE II RULES

Continue to avoid mixing bad carbohydrates with lipids. If you cannot avoid it, try to eat only the minimum and accompanying the item with plenty of fibre (a salad, for example).

Never consume sugar cubes, granulated sugar, honey, jam or sweets. Go on using an artificial sweetener if you find it necessary.

If you eat bad carbohydrates, even occasionally, do so only in small quantities.

Carry on introducing pulses and whole grains into your diet.

Try to eat bread only at breakfast. If need be, eat a little wholemeal bread with your cheese.

Beware of sauces. Make sure they do not contain any flour.

Whenever possible, substitute sunflower margarine for butter, especially at breakfast.

Drink no milk other than skimmed.

Eat more fish and choose " good " lipids in order to protect yourself against cardiovascular disease.

Be careful with desserts containing sugar. However, do not be afraid to eat strawberries, raspberries and blackberries.

You can eat chocolate, sorbets, ice-cream and whipped cream in moderation.

Try to avoid pastries containing flour, fats or sugar.

Choose instead mousses made from fruit and eggs or desserts low in sugar, such as egg custards.

Drink as little as possible at meals.

Never drink alcohol on an empty stomach.

141

Avoid apéritifs and digestifs. These are for exceptional consumption only.

As an apéritif, preferably drink champagne or wine, but first nibble crudités, cooked meats or crabsticks.

With meals, preferably drink water (still) *or wine* (within recognised safe limits).

Do not drink water and wine at the same meal.

Drink water between meals (about a litre and a half a day).

At meals, wait until you have eaten a bit before you start on your wine.

Never drink fizzy drinks, coke or other soft drinks.

Stick to decaffeinated coffee, or weak tea or coffee.

Spread your dietary discrepancies in a balanced way over several meals.

EXAMPLES OF DAILY MENUS FOR PHASE II

Maintaining a stable weight
and balancing the discrepancies

Day 1

Breakfast	Fruit Stoneground wholemeal bread + fruit preserve Low-fat margarine spread * Decaffeinated coffee Skimmed milk
Lunch	Avocado with vinaigrette Steak with French beans Crème caramel To drink : 2 glasses wine *
Evening meal	Vegetable soup Mushroom omelette Green salad Strained fromage frais

---

* slight discrepancy

Day 2

Breakfast

Orange juice
Croissants, brioches **
Butter
Coffee + milk *

Lunch

Crudités (tomato and cucumber)
Grilled fillet of hake
Spinach
Cheese

To drink : 1 glass wine only

Evening meal

Artichokes with vinaigrette
Scrambled eggs with tomato
Green salad

To drink : water

Day 3

Breakfast

Fruit
Stoneground wholemeal bread
Low-fat margarine *
Decaffeinated coffee
Skimmed milk

Lunch

Apéritif : cocktail cheeses + 1 glass
    white wine *

** significant discrepancy
 * minor discrepancy

144

Smoked salmon
Roast leg of lamb with flageolet beans *
Green salad
Cheese
Chocolate mousse *

To drink : 3 glasses wine **

Evening meal	Vegetable soup Stuffed tomatoes (see recipe in Appendix 4) Green salad " Very low fat " fromage frais To drink : water

Day 4

Breakfast	Scrambled eggs Bacon Sausage Decaffeinated coffee + milk
Lunch	1 dozen oysters Grilled tuna with tomato Strawberry tart ** To drink : 2 glasses wine *
Evening meal	Vegetable soup Cauliflower gratin

Green salad
Yogurt

To drink : water

Day 5 (major discrepancy)

Breakfast   Orange juice
                     Cereal or " very low fat " fromage
                        frais
                     Coffee or decaffeinated coffee
                        + skimmed milk

Lunch   Foie gras *
                     Grilled salmon with spinach
                     Bitter chocolate fondant **

                     To drink : 3 glasses wine **

Evening meal   Cheese soufflé
                     Petit salé (salt pork) with lentils **
                     Cheese
                     Œufs à la neige *

                     To drink : 3 glasses wine **

*Note :   Day 5's menu is given only as an example.   It is on no account to
be taken as a recommendation, particularly in the excessive amount of
wine (six glasses being a good deal more than the half-bottle regarded as
the maximum to consume in a day).   This scale of discrepancy should
be considered quite exceptional.*

Day 6 — Full compensatory return to Phase I

Breakfast   Wholemeal bread
" Very low fat " fromage frais
Coffee or decaffeinated coffee
+ skimmed milk

Lunch   Crudités (cucumber, mushrooms, radishes)
Poached hake in tomato sauce
Cheese
To drink : water, tea or herbal tea.

Evening meal   Vegetable soup
Ham
Green salad
1 yogurt

Day 7

Breakfast   Stoneground wholemeal bread
Fromage frais
Coffee or decaffeinated coffee
Skimmed milk

Lunch   Chicory salad
Entrecôte with French beans
Strawberries
To drink : 1 glass wine *

147

Evening meal	Fruit :
	1 orange
	1 apple
	1 pear
	150g strawberries
	To drink : water

Day 8

Breakfast	Stoneground wholemeal bread
	Low-fat margarine *
	Coffee or decaffeinated coffee
	Skimmed milk

Lunch	Prawn cocktail
	Tuna with aubergines
	Green salad
	Cheese
	To drink : 2 glasses wine

Evening meal	Vegetable soup
	Dish made with lentils
	Strawberries
	To drink : 1 glass wine *

CHAPTER VI

HYPOGLYCAEMIA
THE DISEASE OF THE CENTURY

As we have already established, the metabolic process is the means by which the body converts ingested foods into elements vital for its needs. So when, for example, we talk of the metabolism of lipids, we mean the process by which fats are converted within the body.

The main theme of this book comes down to a discussion of the metabolism of carbohydrates and its consequences.

We have seen in earlier chapters how insulin (a hormone secreted by the pancreas) plays a crucial role in the metabolism of carbohydrates. The basic function of insulin is to act upon the glucose in the bloodstream in such a way that the glucose can be absorbed into the body's cells, thus becoming available as fuel to ensure proper functioning of the various organs. Glucose is responsible for the formation of glycogen in the muscles and liver and its presence can sometimes result in the formation of body fat.

In performing its function, the insulin removes

glucose from the bloodstream, so reducing the blood glucose level.

If insulin is secreted by the pancreas too frequently or in excessive amounts — in other words, if it is disproportionate to the amount of glucose to be metabolised — then the glucose in the blood will fall to an abnormally low level. When this happens, you are said to be in a state of hypoglycaemia.

So hypoglycaemia is not necessarily the result of an insufficiency of sugar in the diet, but of over-secretion of insulin. This can arise from previous over-consumption of sugar.

If, for example, you suddenly feel tired at around eleven o'clock in the morning, that generally means that your blood glucose level is below normal. You are in a state of hypoglycaemia.

If you then ingest bad carbohydrate in the form of a biscuit or a sweet snack, this will quickly be metabolised into glucose, your blood glucose level will rise and you will feel suitably restored. But the presence of the glucose in your blood will automatically trigger the production of insulin, which in turn will dispatch the glucose and leave you back in your hypoglycaemic state, only with your blood sugar level now even lower than before. This is the pattern which leads you into the vicious circle of sugar addiction.

Many researchers have even suggested that chronic hypoglycaemia could be a cause of alcoholism. When an alcoholic's blood glucose level dips, he feels bad and senses that he needs a drink. The alcohol is rapidly metabolised, his blood glucose level rises and he feels immeasurably better. Unfortunately, though, the illusion of well-being quickly disappears as the insulin forces his blood glucose level down even further.

Within minutes of his first drink, the alcoholic feels an even greater need for another one to dispel — if only for a short while — the unbearable effects of the hypoglycaemia. When looked at like this, the craving becomes easy to understand.

Adolescents who are heavy consumers of sweet soft drinks have a blood sugar graph which zig-zags up and down very like that of the alcoholic. This is why some American doctors have suggested that consumption of soft drinks can predispose young people to alcoholism, which is becoming an increasingly serious problem on American university campuses. It seems the young person's body is ready and almost conditioned to take the short step from lemonade to alcohol. This is yet another good reason to draw parents' attention to the potential risks of addiction to certain bad carbohydrates.

The symptoms of hypoglycaemia are as follows :

— *tiredness, suddenly " running out of steam "*
— *irritability*
— *nervousness*
— *aggression*
— *impatience*
— *anxiety*
— *yawning, loss of concentration*
— *headaches*
— *excessive perspiration*
— *sweaty palms*
— *learning difficulties*
— *indigestion*

— *nausea*

— *incoherence*

The above list is not exhaustive, but even so it is quite impressive. However, if you are hypoglycaemic it does not mean you will have all these symptoms, nor that the ones you do experience are permanent. Some are, in fact, quite transient and disappear as soon as you eat something. You have probably noticed how some people become progressively more nervous and less equable, or even seem more aggressive, as their normal mealtime approaches.

Among the symptoms of hypoglycaemia, if there is one which crops up more often than the others, as you will probably have noticed in yourself and in those around you, it is *tiredness*.

Indeed, chronic fatigue is so widespread these days that it has come to be a characteristic of the society we live in.

The more people sleep, the more leisure time they have, the more holidays they take, the more tired they seem to become. When they get up in the morning, they feel " whacked " before they start. By the end of the morning they have had enough. After lunch they fall asleep at their desk, as they are hit by post-prandial somnolence. By the end of the afternoon they are having to summon up their last scrap of energy to drag themselves off home. They spend the evening doing nothing, dozing in front of the television. Then at night they are unable to sleep, and when they do drop off it is time to get up... and the cycle begins all over again. So then they blame the stress we have to live with these days, the noise, the pollution or a magnesium deficiency. And all they can think of as a cure is drinking strong coffee, devouring vitamin tablets and mineral capsules or taking up yoga. More often than not, their exhaustion is a blood glucose problem, the product of an unbalanced diet.

These days people's blood glucose level is abnormally low. And this is the direct result of a diet too high in bad carbohydrates. Too much sugar, too many sweet drinks, too much white bread, too many potatoes, too much pasta and rice and too many biscuits, all of which lead to excessive secretion of insulin.

For a long time it was believed that only people who had a tendency to put on weight could suffer from hypoglycaemia. Recent studies, however, particularly some carried out in the past ten years in the United States, have shown that many thin people who consume excessive amounts of sugar and bad carbohydrates are also liable to fall victim to it. The difference lies in their individual metabolism, which decrees that while others put on weight, they do not. But as far as their blood glucose problems are concerned, the same process and the same consequences apply.

Furthermore, these studies show that women are particularly sensitive to variations in their blood glucose level, and it is thought this could account for frequent mood shifts. At all events, it has been shown that postnatal depression is directly linked to the hypoglycaemic state of the woman following childbirth.

If you follow carefully the Method set out in the previous chapter, you will very soon notice that there are other benefits quite apart from weight loss. You will rediscover your *joie de vivre*, your optimism and your vitality. If you used to " run out of steam ", this will cease to be a problem. In fact, you will feel a new person, both mentally and physically.

This is because by eliminating sugar and by cutting down on your consumption of bad carbohydrates you will avoid excessive insulin production and your blood glucose will stabilise at its optimum level. *Little by little your body will go back to following its own instincts, which means producing for itself from its fat reserves whatever sugar it needs.* This is the only way that this optimum blood sugar level can be attained.

Doctors and research scientists I have worked with have assured me that hypoglycaemia is one of the least satisfactorily diagnosed complaints, because its symptoms are so numerous and so varied that GPs rarely spot it. One reason for this could be that very little time is given to the topic during medical training.

But the easiest way to discover whether or not you suffer from hypoglycaemia is to put into practice the eating rules laid down in the previous chapter. Within a week you will be enthusing about how much fitter you feel. You will discover the " inner vitality " that no amount of drinking mineral water had previously been able to persuade to surface.

Many cases of fatigue are linked to a mild deficiency in vitamins or minerals, whether major or trace elements. Low-calorie diet fanatics have a micronutrient deficiency of this kind, on account of their low intake of food. The lack of micronutrients is also exacerbated by agricultural methods which have

154

allowed the land to become overworked and impoverished.

To keep fit, then, it is necessary to eat fruit, vegetables, wholegrains and wholemeal bread and to consume a certain amount of vegetable oil.

You can then be confident you are consuming the right amounts of micronutrients to ensure that your body works at maximum efficiency.

CHAPTER VII

VITAMINS AND MINERALS (MAJOR AND TRACE ELEMENTS)

The modern diet is deficient or at least poor in certain essential nutrients : these are vitamins and minerals, the latter normally being classified as major elements and trace elements. Not only are these substances removed during the refining of foodstuffs, but they tend to be lost in the course of most industrial processes, whether in the production of food or in its conservation.

The consequences of being totally deprived of these nutrients have long been understood. But all the time we are learning more and more about the ill effects caused by relative deficiencies. Two that are worthy of note from our point of view are fatigue and difficulty in losing weight.

VITAMINS

The very word " vitamin " immediately conjures up images of vitality and life.

It is a fact that none of the chemical processes which take place inside us could happen without vitamins. They play a role in the functioning of the hundreds of enzymes which act as biochemical catalysts within the cells of our bodies.

You might logically suppose that in Western countries, where there are no food shortages, we would not be short of vitamins.

And yet the majority of the population is in just that position.

Quite apart from those on low-calorie diets, who cannot extract the nutrients that they need from the limited range of foods they are allowed, the rest of the population also suffers through poor eating habits.

It is well known that high concentrations of vitamins are found in fruit and fibre.

But, according to statistics complied by Professor Cloarec, 37 % of people in France never eat fruit, while 32 % never eat green vegetables.

The situation is all the more critical because these individuals are the very people who also choose to eat highly refined products, such as white flour and white rice, from which, by definition, the vitamins have been removed.

And yet vitamins are essential to the functioning of the human body, even though they are needed in extremely small doses.

But as the body is not capable of synthesising them — that is, manufacturing them for itself — it has to extract them from the daily food intake.

Vitamins may be :

— water-soluble vitamins, which cannot be stored in the body. These are vitamins B and C and niacin. These leach out into the water in which vegetables are cooked, and are lost because the water is not reused to make soup as it was in the old days.

— fat-soluble vitamins, which can be stored. These include in particular vitamins A, D, E and K.

- *Vitamin shortages*

Changes in Western society and the population growth after the Second World War brought with them the phenomena of urbanisation and rural depopulation.

Hand in hand with the necessity of producing more food came the necessity of producing different food, since for the first time in human history the place where food was consumed and the place where it was produced were no longer one and the same.

And so, to boost production levels, intensive farming methods were developed, making use of chemical fertilisers, to say nothing of pesticides, insecticides, herbicides and fungicides.

To overcome the problem of the time it takes to transport foodstuffs to the place of consumption, new conservation techniques were also developed, leading to the generalised use of additives and chemical preserving agents.

All these measures contributed to soils becoming progressively depleted, and led to the foods produced being too full of undesirable chemicals.

And this is why, even before they are harvested, fruit, vegetables and cereals are considerably impoverished in terms of vitamins, and also in terms of trace elements and other mineral salts.

Levels of vitamins A, B1, B2, B3 and C have fallen by over 30 % in certain vegetables because of the way they are grown.

For example, vitamin E has virtually disappeared from lettuce, peas, apples and parsley, just as there is no longer any niacin in strawberries.

As between one crop of spinach and another, variations in vitamin content ranging from 3mg to 150mg per 100g have been recorded.

The nineteenth century fashion for white bread led to research into the refining of flours. The nutritional death-knell for flour was rung in 1875, with the invention of the steel roller mill. Through systematic industrial refining, bread was to be depleted of the greater part of its nutrients : fibre, protein, essential fatty acids, vitamins, minerals and trace elements.

Devoid of all its vital components because of excessive milling, wheat grain has been reduced to hardly more than pure starch, which has nothing more to offer nutritionally than its energy value.

Conversely, the vitamin content of some foods can be increased, though, for example by causing seeds to sprout.

- *The deterioration of vitamins in cooking*

In fruit and vegetables, substantial losses of vitamin C can occur if they are stored for too long, or throught oxidation or cooking.

The greatest losses during cooking result from long, slow cooking at low temperatures. A short cooking time and a high temperature will lead to lower loss. This means that vitamins are better conserved by use of a pressure cooker than in a dish which is left to simmer for hours.

• *Vitamin deficiency through inadequate diet.*

If insufficient food is ingested, as inevitably happens in a low-calorie diet, a vitamin deficiency results.

1500 CALORIE DIET

Vitamins	Percentage of recommended intake
A	30 %
E	60 %
B1	40 %
B2	48 %
B6	49 %
C	45 %
Niacin	43 %
B5	40 %
B9	38 %

• *How to avoid vitamin loss*

— Use the freshest produce you can get, rather than foods which have been on the shelves for days.
— If possible, buy your vegetables on a daily basis, in the market or from your local greengrocer.
— Use as little water as possible in preparation (washing, soaking).
— Choose to eat fruits and vegetables raw (except where this causes indigestion).
— Peel fruit and vegetables as little as possible and make only sparing use of the grater.
— Avoid long, slow cooking.

VITAMIN	SOURCES	DEFICIENCY SYMPTOMS
A (retinol)	Liver, egg yolk, milk, butter, carrots, spinach, tomatoes, apricots	Poor night vision Sensitivity to light Dry skin Skin sensitivity to sunlight Susceptibility to respiratory infections
Provitamin A (beta-carotene)	Carrots, cress, spinach, mango, melon, apricots, broccoli, peaches, butter	
D (calciferol)	Liver, tuna, sardines, egg yolk, mushrooms, butter, cheese Sunshine	In children : rickets In the elderly : osteoporosis and softening of the bones (decalcification)
E (tocopherol)	Oils, hazelnuts, almonds, whole grains, milk, butter, eggs, dark chocolate, wholemeal bread	Muscle fatigue Risk of cardiovascular incidents Aging of skin
K (menadione)	Made by intestinal bacteria Liver, cabbage, spinach, eggs, broccoli, meat, cauliflower	Haemorrhages
B1 (thiamin)	Yeast, wheatgerm, pork, offal, fish, whole grains, wholemeal bread	Fatigue, irritability Loss of recall Loss of appetite, depression, muscle weakness
B2 (riboflavin)	Yeast, liver, kidneys, cheese, almonds, eggs, fish, milk, cocoa	Seborrhea Acne rosacea Photophobia Brittle, lifeless hair Lip and tongue sores, stomatitis
Niacin (nicotinic acid, B3)	Yeast, bran, liver, meat, kidneys, fish, wholemeal bread, dates, pulses Intestinal flora	Fatigue Insomnia Anorexia Depression Skin and mucous membrane lesions

VITAMIN	SOURCES	DEFICIENCY SYMPTOMS
B5 (pantothenic acid)	Yeast, liver, kidneys, eggs, meat, mushrooms, cereals, pulses	Fatigue, headaches Nausea Vomiting Psychoses Low blood pressure Postural problems Hair loss
B6 (pyridoxine)	Yeast, wheat germ, soya, liver, kidneys, meat, fish, wholegrain rice, avocado, pulses, wholemeal bread	Fatigue Depression Irritability Dizziness Nausea Skin lesions Craving for sweet things Headaches due to glutamates
B8 (biotin)	Intestinal flora Yeast, liver, kidneys, chocolate, eggs, mushrooms, chicken, cauliflower, pulses, meat, wholemeal bread	Fatigue, loss of appetite Nausea, muscle fatigue Greasy skin Hair loss Insomnia, depression Neurological problems
B9 (folic acid)	Yeast, liver, oysters, soya, spinach, cress, green vegetables, pulses, wholemeal bread, cheese, milk, wheatgerm	Fatigue Loss of recall Insomnia, depression Mental confusion (in the elderly) Slow healing Neurological problems
B12 (cyanocobal-amine)	Liver, kidneys, oysters, herrings, fish, meat, eggs	Fatigue, irritability Paleness Anaemia, loss of appetite Sleep disorders Neuromuscular aches Loss of recall Depression
C (ascorbic acid)	Rosehips, blackcurrant, parsley, kiwis, broccoli, green vegetables, citrus fruits, liver, kidneys	Fatigue, drowsiness Loss of appetite Muscular aches Lowered resistance to infection Breathlessness on exertion

— Avoid keeping food warm for too long.

— Keep cooking water to use in soup; it contains water-soluble vitamins.

— It is preferable to cook vegetables in steam rather than water.

— Organise your cooking so as not to have left-overs to refrigerate and heat up.

— Choose quality over quantity, selecting organically grown items where possible.

— Roasting or grilling meat retains the most vitamins.

— Frozen foods are richer in vitamins than tinned ones.

— Keep milk away from light.

MINERALS : MAJOR ELEMENTS AND TRACE ELEMENTS

The human body is continuously subject to a large number of chemical reactions. These could not take place without the presence of minerals, both major and trace elements, which act indirectly via the enzymes.

For example, the transmission of nerve impulses depends upon the presence of sodium and potassium. Muscle contraction could not take place without calcium, and the thyroid gland could not produce its hormones without iodine. Similarly, oxygen could not be carried in the blood in the absence of iron, and glucose could not be properly assimilated without chromium.

164

These micronutrients can be placed in two categories :

— Major elements such as calcium, potassium, sodium and sulphur.

— Trace elements, such as chromium, cobalt, zinc, copper, and selenium, which need to be present in extremely small quantities.

A shortage of major elements or trace elements can have a slowing-down effect on the body. It is known, for example, that :

— a manganese deficiency can result in a tendency to hypoglycaemia.

— a deficiency of nickel, chromium or zinc prolongs insulin resistance.

You might think that a deficiency in micronutrients arising from poor eating habits could easily be compensated for by taking supplements in tablet or capsule form. The trouble is that, even though these synthetic products can be of help in cases of serious deficiency, they are not very well absorbed in the intestine.

It is therefore better to aim for a normal, varied diet, containing such quantities of all the major and trace elements as the body may need.

This is why the consumption of fruit, vegetables, raw foods, pulses and whole grains is to be encouraged.

The only supplement worth advocating is a daily intake of brewer's yeast and wheatgerm, as these contain nutrients not easily found elsewhere in our modern diet.

Moreover, brewer's yeast is rich in chromium, which helps raise glucose tolerance, in turn resulting in lower blood glucose and a lower level of blood insulin.

CONTENT PER 100 g	BREWER'S YEAST	WHEATGERM
Water	6 g	11 g
Protein	42 g	26 g
Carbohydrate	19 g	34 g
Lipids	2 g	10 g
Fibre	22 g	17 g
Potassium	1 800 mg	850 mg
Magnesium	230 mg	260 mg
Phosphorus	1 700 mg	1 100 mg
Calcium	100 mg	70 mg
Iron	18 mg	9 mg
Beta-carotene	0,01 mg	0 mg
Vitamin B1	10 mg	2 mg
Vitamin B2	5 mg	0,7 mg
Vitamin B5	12 mg	1,7 mg
Vitamin B6	4 mg	3 mg
Vitamin B12	0,01 mg	0 mg
Folio acid	4 mg	430 mg
Niacin	46 mg	4,5 mg
Vitamin E	0 mg	21 mg

166

CHAPTER VIII

HIGH BLOOD CHOLESTEROL CARDIOVASCULAR DISEASE AND DIET

The main aims of this book arc, firstly, to help you change your eating habits so as to lose any excess weight and, secondly, to show you how to stabilise your weight at its new level while eating an unrestricted choice of foods.

In the previous chapters we saw that the consumption of fats only led to the accumulation of body fat if they were ingested alongside carbohydrates, particularly bad carbohydrates.

This might lead some people to think that they could eat with impunity as much fatty food as they liked, just as long as the fats were not part of a forbidden combination of foods.

Of course, you can do no such thing, as we have taken care to point out at every opportunity.

Changing your eating habits in order to slim is fine, but it is also important that you should be doing it with your health in mind, with an improvement in your fitness being at very least a secondary aim.

I have been taken to task for failing to discuss

cholesterol in the first edition of this book. Indeed, I had set out to do so and had contacted a number of specialists. The trouble was that they all adhered firmly to different views, and as I am not a medical man myself, it did not seem logical to single out one viewpoint. Personal experience, though, had led me to form my own opinion on the subject.

Now, five years on, there is some consensus on the subject of cholesterol and an impressive number of publications on it have appeared.

Furthermore, cholesterol has become one of the major preoccupations of our time, given its role in cardiovascular disease. It is therefore important to offer some comment here.

CHOLESTEROL HAS ITS PLACE

Cholesterol is not some unwelcome intruder. It is actually a substance essential to the formation of certain hormones. The body contains about 100g of it, distributed around the tissues of the nervous system, in the nerves and various other cells.

It is largely synthesised within the body (70 % is accounted for in this way); in particular, 800mg to 1200mg per day is released into the small intestine in the bile.

The cholesterol we are usually concerned with is the cholesterol which is dietary in origin, even though this only amounts to about 30 % of the total in our bodies.

GOOD AND BAD CHOLESTEROL

Cholesterol is not found in isolation in the blood. It is attached to proteins, of which there are two types :

— *low-density lipoproteins* or LDLs, which distribute cholesterol to different cells, notably to those on the artery walls, which then become the site of fatty deposits.

So LDL cholesterol has been christened " bad cholesterol ", because it ends up covering the walls of the blood vessels and clogging the vessels.

The obstruction of the arteries in this way can lead to a cardiovascular incident, such as

- inflammation of the arteries in the lower limbs
- angina or a myocardial infarction
- a cerebrovascular incident (stroke) which may result in paralysis.

— *high-density lipoproteins* or HDLs, which transport cholesterol to the liver, so that it can be eliminated.

HDL cholesterol has been called " good cholesterol ", because it does not lead to arterial deposits. On the contrary, it has the property of cleaning out the atheromatous deposits from the arteries. So it is evident that the higher the level of HDL, the lower the risk of cardiovascular disease.

BLOOD CHOLESTEROL LEVELS

The recommended levels are now much more rigorous than they were in the past. Three measurements are involved :
— total cholesterol (HDL + LDL) should be not higher than 2g per litre of blood.
— LDL cholesterol should be below 1.3g per litre.
— HDL cholesterol should be above 0.45g per litre in a man, and above 0.55g per litre in a woman.

CARDIOVASCULAR RISK FACTORS

The risk of cardiovascular disease is doubled if the total cholesterol level is more than 2.2g per litre of blood, and quadrupled if it is above 2.6g per litre.

However, it has been calculated that 15 % of heart attacks occur in people with a total blood cholesterol level of under 2g per litre. The importance of the total level of cholesterol is therefore only relative.

What is more important is the respective amounts of LDL and HDL present and, above all, the ratio of LDL to total blood cholesterol. It is imperative to keep this ratio below 4:5.

In France, 45 % of adults have blood cholesterol levels above these norms and about 8 million people there have levels above 2.5g per litre. When you consider that bringing down blood cholesterol by 12.5 % reduces the risk of heart attack by 19 %, these figures deserve to be taken seriously.

170

TREATING HIGH BLOOD CHOLESTEROL BY DIET

In cases of high blood cholesterol, the doctor may prescribe medication, but this should be considered a last resort.

In most cases, good dietary management should be all that is needed.

So here is some advice for you to follow, either to bring down your blood cholesterol level if it is too high, or to ward off future problems.

1. Lose some weight

It has been observed that, in most cases, losing some weight brings improvements on all biological fronts. A lower blood cholesterol level is certainly one of the first of these improvements to show up, always provided the subject has not fallen into the error of consuming excessive amounts of bad lipids.

2. Cut down on dietary cholesterol

Foods contain varying amounts of cholesterol. Egg yolks, offal and brewer's yeast contain a great deal.

For a long time, the World Health Organisation recommended a daily intake not in excess of 300mg.

Recent studies, though, have indicated that, surprisingly, this aspect of the diet was of only secondary importance. Raising the daily intake of cholesterol to 1000mg only led to a rise of about 5% in blood cholesterol level.

So one does not need to worry too much about the

sheer overall quantity of cholesterol in foods. What matters, though, is to take account of the extent to which the fatty acids ingested are saturated ones.

3. Know how to choose your lipids

We saw under the classification of foods in Chapter II that fats can be placed in one of three categories.

— *saturated fats,* which are found in meat, cooked meats, poultry, eggs, milk, milk products and cheese.

These fats add to the total blood cholesterol level, and especially to the level of LDL cholesterol, which is deposited on the arterial walls, predisposing the individual to cardiovascular disease.

Recent publications, however, show that eggs and fermented cheeses seem to have a much less marked effect than had been thought.

As for poultry, if the skin is removed it is low in saturated fat. So eating poultry need have little adverse effect on the blood cholesterol level.

— *polyunsaturated fatty acids of animal origin*

These are essentially the fatty acids contained in fish oils. It was long thought that the Eskimos, whose diet is 98 % fish oils, owed their apparent immunity to cardiovascular disease to genetic factors. It was later realised, though, that it was precisely the nature of their diet which was the major factor conferring protection on them.

The consumption of fish oils does indeed lead to a substantial drop in the level of triglycerides and protects against thromboses.

So you can see that, contrary to what was long believed, the fattier the fish the more beneficial it is from the cardiovascular point of view. Eating salmon, tuna, sardines, mackerel, anchovies and herrings is to be encouraged.

— *monounsaturated fatty acids*

Chief amongst these is oleic acid, which is found notably in olive oil.

Olive oil can be said to emerge as the supreme champion among fats which have a beneficial effect on blood cholesterol. It is, in fact, the only one which manages not only to bring down the level of bad cholesterol (LDL), but also to raise the level of the good sort (HDL).

There are those that claim that tuna in olive oil is a passport to a life free of circulatory problems.

4. Increase the amount of fibre in your diet

The presence of fibre in the digestive tract makes for more efficient metabolising of fats.

It has been observed, in particular, that consuming pectin (by eating apples) leads to a significant lowering of the blood cholesterol level. The same has been shown to be true for other soluble fibres, found in oats and pulses (haricot beans, lentils).

5. Cut down on coffee drinking

Studies carried out in the United States and in Norway found that coffee drunk in excess of six cups per day produced a clear rise in overall cholesterol levels and a slight drop in HDL levels. This negative effect was not due to the caffeine, so drinking decaffeinated coffee is not a better option.

6. A little wine will do no harm

Indeed, Professor Masquelier has isolated a molecule present in wine, called procyanidin, which has the advantage of bringing down the total cholesterol level and raising the level of HDL cholesterol.

It also contains polyphenols, which protect the artery walls.

The region of Europe where there is the least cardiovascular disease is Crete, where people drink wine and consume a great deal of olive oil.

This does not mean that it is wise to drink more than three glasses a day of a wine high in tannin.

7. Polish up your lifestyle

Stress, smoking and a sedentary lifestyle also have a negative effect on your cholesterol level. Improving your lifestyle is imperative, not only to cure existing problems, but also to prevent problems arising.

SUMMARY OF ACTION TO REDUCE HIGH BLOOD CHOLESTEROL

— Lose weight, if you are overweight.
— Cut down your meat consumption (maximum 150g per day).
— Choose lean meats, such as venison or lean beef.
— Replace meat on some occasions with poultry (without skin).
— Avoid cooked meats and offal.
— Eat more fish (at least 300g a week).

— Eat very little butter (maximum 10g per day).

— Cut down on cheese.

— Use skimmed milk and "very low fat" milk products.

— Increase your consumption of fibre (fruit, cereals, vegetables, pulses).

— Step up your consumption of monounsaturated and polyunsaturated fatty acids of vegetable origin (olive, sunflower and rapeseed oils).

— Make sure you get enough vitamin A, vitamin E, selenium and chromium (take brewer's yeast and wheatgerm).

— Do not drink too much coffee.

— Drink high-tannin wine if you want to (maximum half a bottle a day).

— Control your stress level.

— Consider taking up an endurance sport.

— Stop smoking.

CHAPTER IX

SUGAR IS A POISON

Sugar is a poison! The ravages it has caused in the twentieth century are as serious as those of alcohol and tobacco put together. That is well-known. It is condemned by doctors the world over. Wherever there is a conference of paediatricians, cardiologists, psychiatrists or dentists, there is talk of the dangers of sugar and, in particular, the dangers of a level of sugar consumption which is rocketing.

In Antiquity sugar, as we know it, barely existed. The Greeks did not even have a word for it.

Round about 325 BC, Alexander the Great, who had pushed his conquests as far as the plains of the Indus, described sugar as " a sort of honey found in the canes and reeds growing by the water ".

Pliny the Elder, in the first century AD, also talked of " the honey from the cane ".

It was not until the time of Nero that the word saccharum was used to denote this exotic product.

In the seventh century AD, sugar began to be cultivated in Persia and in Sicily, and little by little the Arab countries also acquired a taste for it.

A German scholar by the name of Doctor Rauwolf noted in his journal in 1573 that : " Since they have been eating sugar, the Turks and the Moors are no longer the intrepid warriors they once were ".

It was, in fact, through the Crusades that cane sugar became known in Western Europe. And it was not long after this date that sugar also began to be cultivated in the southern part of the Iberian peninsula.

With the conquest of the New World and the expansion of three-way trade, sugar took on an important economic role. Portugal, Spain and England grew rich trading the raw material for slaves, who were in turn put to work in the sugar plantations. By 1700, France too had built a number of refineries.

Napoleon's defeat at Trafalgar in 1805 and the continental blockade which followed led him to disregard the advice of the scientists of the day, and seek ways of producing sugar from beet. This only became truly feasible in 1812, when Benjamin Delessert invented a procedure for extracting the sugar.

By just a few decades later, there was overproduction of sugar in France, though the degree of consumption was still a long way off the level we know today.

In 1880, annual sugar consumption stood at 8kg per person [1], the equivalent of about five lumps of sugar a day. Twenty years later, in 1900, it had more than doubled to 17kg. By 1960, it had reached 30kg and by 1972, was 38kg.

So over the course of two hundred years the average French person's consumption of sugar had risen from less than a kilogram a year to almost 40kg.

In three million years, human beings had never

178

before made such a drastic change to their eating habits in such a short space of time.

And yet the French are by no means the worst affected. In English-speaking countries the situation is even more dramatic, especially in the United States, where the average person consumes about 63kg of sugar a year. And the latest statistics show that, despite all warnings, the graph is still rising[1]. Britain is not so very far behind, with an annual consumption of around 45kg per head.

The most worrying factor of all, though, must be that the proportion of " hidden sugar "[2] shown in the statistics is rising even more rapidly. In 1970, the proportion of sugar intake that was ingested indirectly (in drinks, sweets, preserves and so on) was 58 %. By 1975, that figure had already risen to 63 %.

Indeed, the overall statistics can be misleading. For, with the introduction of artificial sweeteners and under pressure from the medical profession, the direct consumption of sugar (in granulated or lump form) has tended to level off, or even fall.

By contrast, as we have already indicated, the rate of indirect sugar consumption is real cause for alarm, the more so because it affects children and adolescents particularly badly. A 150ml glass of lemonade or coke contains the equivalent of four lumps of sugar.

---

1. One century earlier, in 1789, it had been at the much lower figure of 1kg per head per year.

1. This is not true for France, however, where strenuous efforts have been made in recent years. In 1978 consumption had fallen to 37kg per head, and it is to be hoped this reduction is part of a continuing trend.

2. Hidden sugar is the sugar added to commercially available drinks and foods.

Furthermore, the colder the drink, the less its sweetness is apparent.

Sweetened soft drinks these days form part of most people's diet. The manufacturers are powerful multinational companies and their advertising power is phenomenal. It is quite frightening to see how they have even been able to insinuate themselves into developing countries, where all too often even the basic nutritional needs of the population are not being met.

With more widespread ownership of domestic freezers, ice-creams and other frozen desserts are no longer treats for special occasions, but everyday items. Vending machines in all kinds of public places constitute a permanent temptation to eat sweets. And to make matters worse, these sweet things are cheap enough to be widely accessible. In supermarkets everywhere you can buy a large bag of sweets for pence rather than pounds. The potential customer is perpetually targeted by the ever-present advertising, so that turning away from such blandishments demands nothing short of pure heroism.

It will not come as news to you that sugar is responsible for a large number of diseases. It is one of those things everybody seems to know, but which appears to have no effect on our eating habits, and even less on our children's.

Sugar is the prime culprit in cardiovascular disease. Doctor Yudkin quotes the example of the Massai and Samburu tribes in East Africa, whose diet is very rich in fats but almost devoid of sugar. Coronary illnesses are almost unheard of in these tribes. By contrast, the inhabitants of the island of

Saint Helena, who eat a great deal of sugar but very little fat, have a very high incidence of heart disease.

Dental decay, which is linked to excessive sugar consumption, is so widespread in Western countries that the WHO[1] ranks dental and oral disease third in importance, after cardiovascular disease and cancer, among health problems affecting the industrialised nations.

When we associate sugar and disease, diabetes naturally comes to mind. We are wrong if we believe this problem is purely an inherited one. Of course, not all adult diabetics are overweight, but most are.

Studies have shown that excessive sugar consumption is also a factor in a number of mental illnesses.

And, in any case, in the light of the preceding chapters you will now understand how sugar, a purely chemical product, can cause hypoglycaemia, be responsible for generally upsetting the metabolism and lead to any number of digestive problems.

Finally, to round off this catalogue of disasters, sugar can also lead to vitamin B deficiency. Vitamin B is needed in large quantities for the assimilation of carbohydrates, but sugar, in company with all the refined starches (white flour, white rice, etc.), contains none at all. The body is therefore forced to draw on its vitamin B reserves, resulting in a deficiency whose consequences can include nervous exhaustion, fatigue and depression, as well as loss of concentration, memory and perceptive acuity.

This is an area which could profitably be explored in

---

1. WHO : World Health Organisation.

cases of children experiencing problems with school work.

ARTIFICIAL SWEETENERS

I have advised you to cut out sugar entirely. Obviously, this is impossible to do when it is hidden, as it is, for example, in desserts. But if you can manage to give up granulated and lump sugar, you will already have taken a great step forward.

So you must do one of two things : either do without, or replace it with an artificial sweetener.

There are four main types of artificial sweetener. None, except the poloyols, has any energy value, so nutritionally they are of no interest whatever.

1. Saccharine

Saccharine, discovered in 1879, is the oldest of the sugar substitutes. It is not absorbed by the human body at all, and is 350 times sweeter than the sucrose of normal sugar. Some saccharines have the advantages of being very stable in an acidic medium and of tolerating moderately high temperatures. It was the commonest sweetener before the discovery of aspartame.

2. Cyclamates

These are less widespread, even though their discovery goes back to 1937. They are synthesised from benzine, are less sweet than saccharine and are sometimes accused of leaving an unpleasant after-taste.

However, cyclamates do have the advantage of being completely thermostable; that is, they will stand up to very high temperatures. The most commonly used is sodium cyclamate, but calcium cyclamate and cyclamatic acid are also found.

3. Aspartame

Aspartame was discovered in 1965 in Chicago by James Schlatter, a research scientist for Searle Laboratories.

It is the product of two naturally occurring amino acids, aspartic acid and phenylalanine.

It is 180 to 200 times sweeter than sucrose. It has no bitter after-taste and it is not considered to taste " artificial ".

Over 60 countries now use aspartame in the manufacture of food products and drinks.

Artificial sweeteners have been a controversial topic for many years.

Saccharine in particular was for a long time suspected of being a carcinogen. In the event, however, it seems that it has no toxic effect when taken in daily doses of less than 2.5mg per kilo of body weight, which is equivalent to an adult consuming 60-80 kilograms of sugar. Some countries, like Canada, have banned its use though.

Cyclamates have similarly come under suspicion and in 1969 were banned in the United States.

Aspartame too was from the start controversial, but

all the studies done have cleared it of any charge of toxicity, even at high dosage, and its use has been officially endorsed by the United States Food and Drug Administration.

It is obtainable, as " Nutrasweet ", in two forms :

— as tablets which dissolve quickly in both hot and cold liquids.

— in a powdered form, particularly suitable for use in desserts and in cooking.

In tablet form, it has the sweetening power of one 5gm sugar lump and contains 0.07gm of available carbohydrate. One teaspoonful of powder is equivalent in sweetness to the same quantity of granulated sugar and contains 0.5gm of available carbohydrate.

In 1980, the maximum daily dose recommended by the World Health Organisation was 2 tablets per day per kilo of body weight. This would mean that a person weighing nine and a half stone could consume up to 120 tablets a day with no discernable risk of long-term toxicity. This finding was confirmed in 1984 and again in 1987 by the European Community's Scientific Committee on Human Diet.

But a word of caution about artificial sweeteners is in order. Although they have been shown to have no toxic effects, they could in the long term disturb your metabolism. This is because the body detects sweetness and prepares itself to digest carbohydrates, which then fail to materialise.

When you consume a dose of artificial sweetener in the course of the day, any other consumption of carbohydrate that day will result in an a greater than normal rise in blood glucose level, followed by a hypoglycaemic reaction. It is as if the body is " frus-

184

trated " by ingesting the sweetener and makes up for it when it is given carbohydrates by seeing that they are maximally absorbed in the intestine. This raising of the coefficient of absorption of the carbohydrates leads to a greater rise in blood glucose level than would normally be expected with the carbohydrate in question. This in turn leads to a higher amount of insulin being released, resulting in secondary hypoglycaemia. But as hyperinsulinism is a factor in the accumulation of body fat, and as the hypoglycaemia lead to a premature sensation of hunger, one has to wonder whether taking artificial sweeteners does not, indirectly, lead to putting on weight.

From childhood, care needs to be taken not to overencourage a fondness for sweet things, but to enable children to enjoy instead the other basic sensations of taste, appreciating sharp and bitter flavours.

For the " sugar-addicted " child or adolescent, artificially sweetened soft drinks can provide a transition from sugared drinks to water. In the end, though, you must convince yourself that the only suitable drink for a child to consume with main meals is water. At teatime, fresh fruit-juice or milk are vastly preferable to a fizzy drink.

In short, the long-term answer is that the taste buds must be weaned off sweet things, and sweeteners do just the opposite.

So we must be wary of foods which can catch us out by not being what they seem.

This has never been truer than now, when the food industry is busy developing proteins which taste like lipids, designed to replace dietary fats!

Faced with these false signals, our bodies are in danger of not knowing which flavour to turn to!

So then, the use of an artificial sweetener should only be a temporary measure. Your long-term goal should be to wean yourself off the taste of sugar.

4. Polyols

Within the range of "false sugars" we can also include the polyols, or bulk sweeteners, which provide the necessary bulk in certain manufactured products, such as chocolate, chewing-gum and sweets. This is needed because only a very small volume of sweetener actually has to be used to give the desired sweetness.

Unfortunately, the only advantage of polyols over sugar is that they do not encourage tooth decay. They have almost the same energy value as sugar and release fatty acids to be absorbed in the colon. Their glycaemic index varies from 25 to 65. Because they can ferment in the colon, they can also lead to bloating and diarrhoea.

This means that, contrary to what we are often told, the use of these substances cannot prevent you putting on weight, and even less can they help you to slim.

The words "contains no sugar" on a label often disguises the presence of polyols : sorbitol, mannitol, xylitol, maltitol, lactitol, lycasin, polydextrose, and so on.

CHAPTER X

HOW TO FLATTEN
YOUR STOMACH

The vast majority of women worry about their weight, and women generally tend to be concerned at the common problem of a " tummy " which is not always as flat as they would like.

A woman's abdomen is a particularly elastic and sensitive area of her body.

She may be understandably concerned over what she feels are unsightly variations in her size that are the result of the physiological activity taking place inside her.

Most of the time a distended abdomen is put down to the functioning of the reproductive system. Certainly, as we have already mentioned, a woman tends to be prone to fluid retention just before her period. But, although it may be most noticeable in the legs and pelvic area, the fluid retained is to an extent distributed around the body. By contrast, the typically female distribution of body fat around the pelvis and thighs has a physical function, in that it is designed to constitute an energy reserve which will ensure that the woman can breastfeed, even at a time of scarcity such as the human race has experienced through the millennia.

Fluid retention is not, in itself, a sufficient explanation for a permanently distended abdomen.

The bloating is neither more nor less than the sign of chronic digestive problems linked to poor eating habits.

From sections of this book which discuss the technicalities of digestion, you will have realised that, even if particular bad food combinations do not actually lead to accumulation of body fat, they will be at the root of digestive problems.

You will have realised, of course, that we cannot lay at the door of bad food combinations the entire blame for the (sometimes serious) disorders we have listed. The point I have tried to make is that where one of these illnesses does crop up, its cause is very probably closely linked to consuming inappropriate combinations of foods.

Whether or not you have weight to lose, if you are a woman and tend to have a " tummy " you need to follow certain of the rules explained in the previous chapters. Let me recap for the sake of those of you who may only be concerned about this particular problem and have not read every other chapter in the book all that carefully. If this applies to you, however, I would stress to you the importance of reading the following chapters :

" Classification of foods "

" Hypoglycaemia "

" Sugar is a poison ".

EAT FRUIT ON AN EMPTY STOMACH

Fruit is excellent for your health, but on one condition; *that it is never eaten long with anything else.*

I have already explained that if fruit — which is generally acid — is mixed with meat, it will lead to serious digestive problems.

Being a victim of such problems, though, does not necessarily mean you are aware of them. Some people, of course, have high sensitivity and very quickly learn what is not for them, because the consequences (abdominal cramps, bilious attacks, diarrhoea) make their presence all too uncomfortably felt.

For most people, however, trouble does not show up in immediate acute symptoms, because the body is good at resisting the damage and taking steps to compensate.

But this does not mean that nothing adverse is happening. The damage is occurring deep down and bides its time before one day producing overt symptoms.

Some individuals suffer unbearable feelings of bloating when they eat fruit at the end of a meal, and naturally, people with such obvious symptoms will have incentive enough to give up the practice of their own accord.

If this does not happen to you, however, you will have had no reason to give up what you thought was a sensible eating habit.

But if your stomach is not at present perfectly flat, one of the causes is likely to be your habit of finishing a meal with fruit.

As we have already discussed, fruit is metabolised very quickly; it is digested within about twenty minutes.

Within a very short time after being ingested, it is already in the small intestine, where it is assimilated. This is where, in particular, the vitamins it contains are absorbed into the body.

You can see, therefore, that if you eat fruit at the end of the meal, the process will be blocked, as the fruit will have to wait its turn, as it were, for its session in the small intestine.

The trouble is that fruit is by nature impatient, and is not prepared to tolerate without complaint getting stuck in a digestive traffic jam. So, instead of waiting its turn patiently, it starts making its unwelcome presence felt and creating havoc.

First, it degrades to the point of destruction the enzyme medium which is needed — often crucially — for the efficient digestion of the other foods currently in the stomach, and their subsequent smooth passage into the next part of the digestive tract. Production of pepsin, the enzyme essential to the metabolising of meat, will be upset.

So the entire contents of the stomach will be thrown into complete confusion by the gate-crashing arrival of the fruit. The result will be a general slowing-down of the digestive process, with the following conse-quences :

— starches and meats will be insufficiently digested in the stomach. The chemical changes at this stage will be incomplete, making effective digestion at the next stage of the process impossible.

— the fruit, which, by its nature, needs to pass

190

through the stomach very rapidly, will find itself trapped there by the other foods needing slower digestion.

And in this warm, humid environment, the fruit undergoes change. It ferments, because it contains carbohydrates which are rapidly converted into alcohol.

Examples are quoted of people who were great fruit-eaters and who fell victim to cirrhosis of the liver, even though they had not touched a drop of alcohol in their lives. Now you can see how this could happen!

But it is in the small intestine that the worst misfortunes befall, since the " goods " delivered from the stomach do not match up with their delivery note, and for good reason. The meat will have been incompletely digested in the stomach and the fruit, totally transformed by fermentation, will have lost all its vitamins.

The small intestine is somewhat " thrown " when faced with these " substandard goods ".

It first does its level best to make good the damage. To this end it tries to use what, in metabolic terms, amounts to an emergency procedure. The snag is that once again the digestive process is slowed down.

The small intestine, upset by this, becomes irritated and swollen.

Given a woman's physical sensitivity to such anomalies, when these patterns are repeated again and again the abdomen tends to become progressively more distended.

Disturbances to the digestive process also leave the large intestine having to work extra hard, as it has to accept matter which has not been fully digested. It too has to resort to emergency measures, mainly in order to destroy the food remnants by fermentation or decomposition, depending on the nature of the food-stuff.

The necessity of turning to these emergency measures too frequently, or even as a matter of course, leads to a chronically disordered large intestine, whose normal function is constantly disrupted.

You need seek no further to identify the causes of dysfunction of the colon. At all events, one of the more obvious consequences of these problems is a permanently swollen and bloated abdomen.

HOW SHOULD FRUIT BE EATEN?

As fruit cannot be combined with any other foods without upsetting the digestive process, it is imperative, as I have indicated, to eat it on its own and, above all, on an empty stomach.

Rather than eating fruit at the end of the meal, you should eat the fruit first. Ideally, this should be done a good hour ahead of the meal. But you must be particularly careful to allow time for the previous meal to be completely digested; in other words, wait for about three hours after a main meal.

So there are three points in the day when you can have fruit :

— when you wake up in the morning, at least half an hour before breakfast.

— in the late afternoon (at, say, half past five), at least four hours after you have finished lunch. This assumes you do not have a meal at tea-time, but actually, fruit is an excellent tea-time snack.

— before you go to bed in the evening, as long as you leave about four hours after your evening meal.

Remember that citrus fruits (oranges, grapefruit, clementines) are best avoided before bed, as the vitamin C they contain may stop you sleeping. They are excellent to eat first thing in the morning or as a little pick-me-up in the afternoon.

BEWARE OF FRUIT JUICE!

Real specialists in nutrition tend to grimace when you mention fruit juice. They consider, strange as it may seem, that fruit juice is not a natural drink.

We eat fruit in the belief that it contains excellent nutrients essential to our health, and what we usually have in mind is vitamins and minerals.

There are those who think that by drinking " concentrated fruit " in the form of juice they are absorbing even more vitamins.

Unfortunately, this does not quite hold good, as most of the vitamins present in fruit are destroyed when the fruit is turned into juice. Once they are allowed to escape from the normal environment of the whole fruit, they are extremely short-lived.

To make matters worse, most of the vital part of the fruit remains in the pulp, which is discarded once the juice has been extracted from it.

And finally, once separated from the pulp, the juice quickly acquires a very high level of acidity, which has to be counteracted by adding sugar.

At the risk of surprising you, therefore, I would advise you against fruit juice, even if you make it yourself.

Quite apart from its effect on other foods, fruit juice, just like fruit eaten as part of a meal, will irritate the digestive tract with its acidity; the acidity will also destroy other vitamins, just as vinegar would. At very least, avoid consuming any more fruit juice than you would if you ate the fruit it came from, add a little water and sweeten it with an artificial sweetener.

ACTION POINTS TO ACHIEVE A FLAT STOMACH

If your stomach bulges and you feel permanently bloated, you can regain the flat stomach you had at eighteen by sticking to the following rules :

— *never eat fruit except on an empty stomach.*

— *never mix protein-lipids with carbohydrates.*

— *ban fizzy drinks (beer, mineral water, soft drinks).*

— *do some tummy-toning exercises to improve your muscle tone (a quarter of an hour every morning).*

— *avoid constipation by eating bread which is wholemeal, stoneground wholemeal or contains bran, and plenty of other dietary fibre.*

— *finally, do deep relaxation or yoga exercises.*

Some forms of bloating, such as those caused by swallowing air, cam be partly, if not wholly, nervous in origin.

So relaxation can help you regain your flat stomach, but it will not achieve enough on its own to outweigh the unnatural food combinations you have indulged in up to now.

194

CHAPTER XI

HOW SHOULD WE FEED CHILDREN?

The best way to feed young children, especially infants, is one of every mother's biggest preoccupations. The way in which a baby accepts food in the first few months will determine the child's state of health, and even its chances of survival.

If during this period the child is unwell — off its food or suffering from vomiting, diarrhoea, allergies, and so on — the doctor, in the course of his investigations, will undoubtedly take a close look at the baby's diet and suggest some adjustments to it.

Doctors are acutely aware that, in a very young child, health problems almost always stem from diet. They are much more likely to effect a cure by changing this diet, or fine-tuning it, than by prescribing medication.

By contrast, once a child is older, especially once he has gone on to " normal food ", more or less like an adult's, and is eating some of everything or almost everything, it no longer occurs to either parents or doctors to consider eating habits as a possible cause if the child is unwell.

This really is a pity, because if they did most children's health problems could be resolved.

Illness in a child, as in anyone else, is first of all a sign of some physical weakness or other.

The human body is normally endowed with a natural defence mechanism to fight off all attacks from germs in the environment. When a small child is at the stage of putting everything into its mouth, people often say the infant must be " immune to germs ". The implication is that the child is equipped with natural defences which enable it to fend off attacks from germs.

But it is not just babies who are fortunate enough to have this immune system; the growing child, and indeed the adult, retain the ability to resist infection, and the body makes constant use of this ability in order to survive in its germ-ridden environment.

However, if the body is weakened in some way, the result is that these defences become less efficient, and more open to attack.

Leaving aside viral infections, all other illnesses can be put down to this kind of temporary weakening of the body.

And such a weakening is, in most cases, attributable to dietary problems.

This is why parents should keep a continuing watch on their children's food.

Unfortunately, the food of children in industrialised countries, although not lacking in quantity, leaves more and more to be desired in terms of quality.

In addition, some food combinations are not well tolerated by children and, in some cases, would be better avoided completely.

AN APPALLING DIET

Reflecting on how children are fed these days, I cannot help thinking about how domestic pets are fed.

A few years back, people used to make stew for the dog or food for the cat. Nowadays they open a tin. So much easier!

And we are keen to have pets, as long as we do not have to look after them.

It is yet another illustration of a fundamental characteristic of our society. We want all the advantages without any of the disadvantages. In other words, we want to " have our cake and eat it ".

What more natural, too, than that people should aspire to having children? But these days there is a tendency to want children just as long as they do not take too much looking after.

So that our aspirations can be met, our little darlings have become the object of a sort of organised child-rearing industry built around crèches and child-minders. As, just as in the case of our pets, we have found practical, commercially-available solutions to the question of feeding our kids. You just have to open a tin or a little jar of baby food.

Do not worry, I am not a backwoodsman to the extent of condemning all preserved foods; some are very good. What I am up in arms about, though, is how widespread their use has become.

So here are the principles I recommend for feeding your children. The main aim is to ensure that children enjoy the good health which comes naturally from a healthy diet.

FOODS TO KEEP AN EYE ON

Bread

Children, like adults, should not eat " white " bread — that is, ordinary bread made with refined flours. As I have pointed out elsewhere, naturally occurring minerals, especially magnesium, disappear in the refining process.

Also destroyed by the process is vitamin B. It is known that this vitamin is essential for the metabolising of carbohydrates. Vitamin B deficiency leads to the risk of digestive problems and unnecessary fatigue.

It is sometimes claimed that eating wholemeal bread tends to lead to calcium deficiency. This is untrue, even when the bread contains no yeast. It is rich in minerals and, in any case, will take its place in the child's diet alongside dairy products rich in calcium.

Starchy foods

If the child is of normal weight, which would seem to indicate satisfactory carbohydrate tolerance, there is no reason to cut out starchy foods completely. But this does not mean that the child's diet should be based on them, as is so often the case.

Systematic use of bad carbohydrates, chiefly potatoes, rice and pasta, generally stems from lack of imagination. In point of fact, it is perfectly possible to build variety into meals without incurring extra expense. If you read through the chart in Appendix 2 again, you will see there are quantities of vegetables you just might not think of.

It is imperative that children be taught to eat things other than bad carbohydrates. They may well be able to tolerate them at their age, but this may cease to be the case once they have finished growing. So very early on they must be encouraged to like other foods, particularly the other vegetables we have mentioned.

When it comes to pasta, it would be better if this were made from unrefined flour. Other kinds of pasta should not be included too often because, as with white bread, there is some risk of the habit leading to a vitamin B deficiency.

As for rice, it is best to use wholegrain and to serve it as in the Recipe in Appendix 4. As you know, wholegrain rice in tomato constitutes a complete dish in itself.

Finally, remember that some starchy foods are good carbohydrates. This applies to lentils and dried beans. So have no qualms about including them frequently.

Fruit

The child's body has resources which the adult's has long since lost. The child can metabolise without much apparent difficulty food combinations including fruit.

So there is no harm in continuing to let children eat fruit at the end of a meal.

If, however, there is evidence of any digestive disturbance (bloating, abdominal pain, flatulence), then it would be better to cut out fruit at mealtimes. Fruit will then be eaten, following the adult pattern, on an empty stomach, mainly on getting up in the morning or going to bed at night, or on its own at tea-time.

Drinks

Water is definitely the only drink suitable for children. Anything remotely resembling fizzy drinks, synthetic fruit juices, squashes or colas, must be ruled out at all cost. They amount to nothing short of poison for children.

On rare occasions, such as a birthday or a family gathering, you can let your child drink a few glasses of a soft drink, but keep in mind that it is doing as much harm as if the child were drinking alcohol. In fact, a child drinking cola would actually be better off drinking alcohol.

The squashes and syrups you dilute in water are to be avoided too, as they are very heavily sweetened. By making the child used to sweet flavours, they lead to real addiction.

Milk is not advisable during meals. It is always unwise to drink milk with food, because it curdles in the stomach. The curds then cloak particles of food, preventing the gastric juices from reaching them. So drinking milk at a meal is a sure recipe for indigestion.

Children can drink milk during the day, but it is best to see they do so on an empty stomach.

At breakfast, there is not the same problem. Hot

200

milk is much more easily digested and the difficulties described above do not occur to the same extent.

Sugar and sweet things in general

I would not go so far as to ban sugar completely for children, even though that would be far and away the most rational thing to do. I would, though, counsel a very strict approach to sugar consumption.

Apart from the sugar they have in their breakfast, what they put on their fromage frais or yogurt and what is contained in desserts (puddings, pastries, ice-cream) — and this is already a very great deal — do not allow your children to eat sugar, in whatever form.

On the black list are all forms of sweets, including boiled sweets, fruit pastilles and choc-bars (these can contain almost 80 % sugar).

If you need convincing for good that sugar is a real poison, just reread Chapter IX. Sugar is every bit as serious a threat to children as to adults, if not more so.

Moreover, it is important not to allow the young to become addicted to sweet flavours. This is not only necessary for their health now, but is vital for it in the future.

I know it is difficult to stop children from following consumer trends, when they live in an environment in which they are constant targets. But that is no reason to give up trying, or making out that nothing can be done about it.

What can be done, at least, is to establish a strict regime at home, and to encourage children, from the earliest age, not to get used to the taste of sugar. This is what will prevent them from ending up as slaves to it.

This is why I would disagree with the advice of doctors who advocate giving babies sugared water. They can perfectly well get used to drinking pure water. And if your children are given sweets as presents, try to spirit away most of the packet with a view to removing them from circulation completely later on.

Again, even if the quantity of sweets consumed is modest, eating them before meals must be strictly forbidden. If eaten then, not only does the sugar spoil the appetite, but it will also upset the digestion of what little food the child can still manage.

A final reminder that consuming sugar can lead to a vitamin B deficiency. As we have already stressed, this vitamin is essential to carbohydrate metabolism. A shortage of it in the diet causes the body to draw on its reserves, thus creating a deficiency which may result in *fatigue, difficulty in concentrating, loss of recall* and even a particular form of depression. It is obvious that there is a serious risk the child's school work will suffer.

ARTIFICIAL SWEETENERS RATHER THAN SUGAR FOR CHILDREN?

If it is all right for an adult sometimes to replace sugar with an artificial sweetener, then why should it not be all right for children? It is, indeed, a good question.

If the child is really overweight for his or her age, then it can become necessary to use a sweetener.

If, however, the child is of normal weight, there is no reason to cut out completely the lumps of sugar that are popped into the breakfast drink, or the spoonful of granulated sugar that is stirred into the yogurt[1].

On the other hand, what you can do to restrict the daily sugar intake of children (and, indeed, of the whole family) is to use a sweetener when making desserts.

So with all this in mind, let us now look at how you can organise your child's four meals a day.

MAIN MEALS

The aims to be kept in mind when making up children's menus are as follows :

— *avoid too many bad carbohydrates, so as not to upset the child's metabolism.*

— *avoid unnatural food combinations which weaken the body's defences, leading to a large number of health problems.*

When it comes to nutrition, people will tell you with the kind of total conviction that springs from common sense, that the thing to do is to make up " balanced meals ". This is generally taken to mean meals that contain protein, carbohydrate and fat, all lumped together.

This is a completely erroneous view!

---

1. You can also replace white sugar (sucrose) with fructose, now commercially available, which has a much lower glycaemic index.

It is perfectly true that we need to eat proteins, carbohydrates, fats and fibre in order to be certain of absorbing everything the body needs. And this is particularly important for the growing bodies of children.

But the error commonly propounded, not least by the medical profession, is the belief that all these elements need to be balanced within one meal.

When we talk of balanced meals, we need to add the caveat that *the balance will be achieved over several meals and not within a single meal.* This makes all the difference. And this is the main point which has to be understood and respected if we are to avoid all the metabolic problems we have discussed in the course of this book.

In other words, take care when making meals for your children to see that they are principally protein-lipid or principally carbohydrate. But far from trying to combine the two in the same meal, avoid mixing them at all.

BREAKFAST

There is something to be said for the old British tradition of making breakfast the largest meal of the day. This is particularly true for children. Where the traditional British breakfast goes wrong though, is if it attempts to be a " balanced " meal, including both carbohydrate (cereals, for example) and protein-lipids (eggs, meats).

With children, my advice would be to give them a predominantly *carbohydrate* breakfast.

204

This might contain any mixture of the following :

— bread, preferably wholemeal.
— cereals (wholegrain, if possible, and avoiding those containing puffed rice, maize, sugar, honey or caramel).
— fresh fruit (but it is essential this is eaten first).
— sugar-free fruit preserve.
— semi-skimmed milk products.

To the extent that " good " carbohydrates are the dominant component of this meal, it would be better for the child to consume only skimmed or semi-skimmed milk and vegetable fats (margarine rather than butter).

If the child wants to eat fromage frais or a yogurt, it is essential that these are " very low fat ".

I am definitely against honey or jam, since the concentration of sugar (even the naturally-occurring sugar in honey) is too high. The use of jam must be only very occasional (though sugar-free fruit preserves are excellent).

LUNCH

Lunch will be dominated by *proteins* and *lipids*, so it will inevitably contain either meat or fish.

But ideally the meat or fish will not be regularly served with potatoes, rice or pasta. The accompanying vegetables are better chosen from among French beans, celery, cauliflower, mushrooms or others listed in Appendix 2.

If the main course is based on protein and lipids (meat, fish or cooked meats), it is a good idea to stick to

205

milk products or cheese for the dessert course. The children can eat as much of these as they like.

Unfortunately, children of school age often have their mid-day meal at school, which may mean " school dinners ". If this is so, parents lose some control over the diet of their offspring. But as long as the child is not a " fatty ", this should not be catastrophic. Adjustments can be made to other meals to compensate.

And children who have formed good habits at home, such as not eating bread with main meals and eating fruit on an empty stomach, will of their own accord limit the damage done by school meals.

TEA

For people in general and children in particular it is better to pop in an extra meal than to skip one. Like breakfast, tea will be essentially carbohydrate.

If children eat bread for tea, it should be wholemeal, or made with flour which is not too refined. It can be spread with margarine, but avoid jam.

It is perfectly acceptable to give a child a bar of chocolate, as long as it is good quality chocolate with a high (minimum 60 %) cocoa content.

SUPPER

A child's supper can either be protein-lipid, based on meat, fish or eggs, or else based on " good " carbohydrate of the kind which is a dish in itself : lentils, wholegrain rice or wholewheat pasta.

But whichever of these options you go for, the child's first course should be a thick vegetable soup (leek, tomato, celery, etc.)

Generally speaking, children are reluctant to eat enough green vegetables. These, as you know, provide the dietary fibre so necessary for good intestinal function and are rich in vitamins and minerals. The best way of ensuring children eat vegetables is to use the liquidiser to turn them into a good vegetable soup.

There is a third category of dish which is highly suited to children, and which they love, and that is stuffed vegetables; you can use tomatoes, aubergines, courgettes, artichokes or cabbage.

Stuffed vegetables are a good way of using high-fibre vegetables and certainly ring the changes on the endless old pasta, rice and potato.

At supper, you can give children low-fat dairy products, made with semi-skimmed milk; you can make egg custards and crème caramel with fructose or artificial sweetener instead of sugar.

Come what may, there is one type of food which should not be allowed to enter the house : sandwiches, hamburgers and hot dogs. You cannot stop your children from liking hamburgers, just as you cannot stop them from liking fizzy fruit drinks and colas. But that is not a good enough reason to encourage them to eat these things at home. It is a type of eating which undermines children's health, because it involves too much bad carbohydrate in combination with meat.

So reserve this kind of food for the odd occasion

when it is a convenient way of keeping hunger at bay, such as when you are out for the day. The hot dog and the hamburger were originally invented in America as a quick way of eating, either on the job if there was no proper lunch break or on the long journeys all too common in a vast country like the United States.

Eating a hot dog or a hamburger at home makes about as much sense as sleeping in a sleeping-bag on a four-poster bed. In fact, it is worse, because it puts your health at risk. So do not let laziness lead you into such deplorable behaviour. Sadly, this is just what is done by most people in many so-called civilised countries, to the extent that some children do not even know what a proper meal is.

So take your children to MacDonald's or Burger King once in a while for fun, or for quickness if you are on a journey, but it really must be only once in a while.

SOME SPECIAL CASES

Overweight children

Some children can become overweight very young, without their parents being sufficiently concerned to consult a doctor.

If parents do decide to seek medical advice, though, in most cases the doctor's answer will be that a few extra pounds does not make the child positively obese. He will rightly argue that a low calorie diet is not to be considered for a growing child. Nine times

208

out of ten, he will manage to reassure the parents that when the child is older, particularly when he or she reaches adolescence, normal weight should come of its own accord.

But, in fact, you need to be aware that excess weight in a child is invariably an outward sign of disturbed metabolism.

So take childhood plumpness seriously. If the problem is tackled in time, it will be quite easy to restore the right balance.

In children, as in adults, excess body fat is evidence of poor glucose tolerance. The Method, as set out on Chapter V, should be strictly applied.

When the child returns to normal weight, it will be possible, just as it is with adults, to reintroduce gradually a certain number of bad carbohydrates, which will constitute discrepancies needing to be carefully managed.

It is true that some boys who are overweight gradually lose their plumpness at puberty, without making any dietary changes. At this time an adolescent is going through important physical changes which use up a great deal of energy. And usually this coincides with a period of intense physical activity.

Be careful, though, for an adolescent boy of normal weight who was a fat child will once again be a candidate for overweight on reaching adulthood.

In a girl the situation is usually the other way round. It is around puberty, when her body is changing to that of a woman, that there is a risk of putting on weight. As we have seen in an earlier chapter, the female body is very sensitive and any period of hormonal change (be it puberty, pregnancy or the menopause) constitutes a risk to metabolic harmony.

Girls and women themselves are very aware of this, but many, in an effort to look after their figure, unfortunately resort to diets which leave them dying of hunger and which can but lead to depression.

There is no objection at all to girls who tend to put on weight at puberty following the eating rules in this book. Not only will they find this is good for their figure, but they will also discover a new feeling of vitality which should help them to go out and conquer the world.

The child who is always tired

Does it not strike you how these days more and more children and adolescents are tired and listless, just about fit to drag themselves out of bed and into an armchair?

Remember that an excess of bad carbohydrates at breakfast will lead to hypoglycaemia at about 11 o'clock, and with it sleepiness, lack of concentration, yawning, apathy or aggression — the signs teachers so often notice in their pupils towards the end of the morning.

The phenomenon is likely to be repeated later in the day, if children consume too much potato, too much white bread and too many sweet drinks.

Tea, if it is based on fats and sugars (cakes and biscuits, for example) causes further trouble.

When children get home from school, all too often they sit in front of the television. Not only does this encourage them to nibble at things, but the young, who are impressionable and still learning the skills of critical evaluation, can be persuaded into eating sweets and biscuits. A visit to the sports centre will do them more good than "armchair" sport via the television.

It is important that children should be introduced early to a wide variety of foods, otherwise there is a risk that they will develop a dislike of just the high-fibre foods, such as fruit, vegetables and pulses, which are rich in vitamins and minerals.

Deficiencies in any of these can be another factor contributing to debility.

CHAPTER XII

SLIMMING WITHOUT SPORT

In his song " Tu t'laisses aller " (" You're letting yourself go "), the French singer Charles Aznavour advises his girlfriend, who apparently looks a bit of a scarecrow, to " take up a sport and lose some weight ! "

Yet another misconception. You can tell Aznavour has never had a weight problem, or he would have realised that, contrary to popular belief, *sport has never caused anyone to slim.*

When you first became concerned about your excess weight, I imagine that you, like many others, decided to take up a sport — or go back to one. So maybe you lighted on cycling, or jogging, or possibly both.

Having personally tried both, I can assure you that the results are nil.

Sport is a great way of taking exercise, relaxing, unwinding, getting oxygen into your lungs, meeting friends or just getting out of the house. It has every advantage. Except one — that of making you lose weight. If you stick to the bad eating habits which most people have these days, no amount of sport will make you lose weight.

Exercising to lose weight is rather like the calorie theory; it is based on the same kind of myth. When you take up a sport with a view to slimming, you tend to measure your success by how much sweat you manage to shed.

But what you are losing is water. And even if you are " burning off the calories ", this energy is coming from glycogen, your temporary energy reserves, the ones which are fuelled by your consumption of carbohydrates.

After your first session of vigorous exercise, you may indeed notice (if you have extremely accurate scales) that you have lost a few ounces.

But once you are in the habit of asking your muscles to make this kind of effort regularly — every Saturday, for example — your body will gradually readjust, so that its " supply " meets your " demand ". If your demand then increases, it will simply put aside enough glycogen to meet that new demand.

Very soon you will notice that not only are you not losing weight any more, but are back where you started. You may even find you have put on a little more. Remember the hungry dog that buries its bone. If you ask greater effort of your body, no problem; it will just behave prudently and decide to increase its stocks a little more, just in case. And you are into the downward spiral.

To try and outwit your body, you react by adding five kilometres a week to your cycle ride. But the little computer inside you knows all about supply and demand, and it makes the adjustment.

And that is how, for every couple of ounces lost, you gain a couple more and, at the same time, put your health seriously at risk. In sport the golden rule you must always observe is : " never push the body beyond its limits ". You would not dream of entering for the Le Mans 24 Hour Race in a 2CV. And yet that is just what you are doing when you take on an exercise programme which is too ambitious for your age, your physical condition or your level of training.

So take up sport for all the good reasons which are always quoted, or just for the sheer pleasure of it, but do not rely on it to do anything for your weight problem if you are not also prepared to change your eating habits.

If, however, you adopt the Method described in this book, exercise will help you speed up your slimming in Phase I. But above all, you must understand that this is because the physical effort you put in will be helping to get your metabolic functions back in balance.

In Phase I, your glucose should be provided largely from your body fat. If you increase the demand for glucose, therefore, your fat reserves should disappear more quickly.

It has been observed, too, that physical effort is particularly beneficial for obese people, whose fat cells are resistant to insulin; this leads the pancreas to produce too much of it (hyperinsulinism). In addition, obesity upsets thermogenesis, which means, paradoxically, that the fatter you are the less energy you expend for the same physical effort.

So adopting the eating principles of this Method and taking reasonable exercise can be seen as complementary and, together, they will enable you to achieve a more successful return to normal weight. While over-coming your insulin resistance more quickly, you will also feel more in tune with your body, especially as you regain your more attractive silhouette.

CHAPTER XIII

YOUR IDEAL WEIGHT

When we step on the scales, what exactly are we weighing? The total weight of a body composed of bones, muscles, body fat, organs, gut, nerves and water. Body fat makes up, on average, 15 % of a man's weight and 22 % of a woman's.

Obesity is defined as the presence of 20 % more body fat than the average. But how can we assess the exact quantity of body fat present in a particular individual? One way is to measure the thickness of a fold of skin with callipers, but this does not give a very accurate indication.

We have no alternative to defining obesity in terms of excess weight, although this gives no idea of the relative weights of body fat and of the mass of muscles, organs, and so on.

Rather that relying on the weight tables so rigidly drawn up by American insurance companies, it is simpler to establish something like the notion of an ideal weight using the Lorentz formula (in which height is expressed in centimetres and weight in kilograms) :

$$\text{Weight} = (\text{Height} - 100) - \frac{(\text{Height} - 150)}{4}$$

for a man

$$\text{Weight} = (\text{Height} - 100) - \frac{(\text{Height} - 150)}{2}$$

for a woman

This formula, however, takes no account of age or bone structure.

The internationally recognised formula these days is the Quetelet Index (or BMI, standing for Body Mass Index), which expresses the ratio of the individual's weight to the square of his or her height.

$$\text{Index} = \frac{\text{Weight (in kg)}}{\text{Height} \times \text{Height (in metres)}}$$

An index of 20 to 25 in a man and 19 to 24 in a woman is considered normal. With an index of up to 30 an individual is described as overweight, beyond that as obese. A BMI above 40 indicates severe obesity and cause for medical concern.

This definition is a medical rather than an aesthetic one, but the BMI has the advantage that it correlates well with the proportion of body fat.

A simple way of calculating the index
is to use the following table :

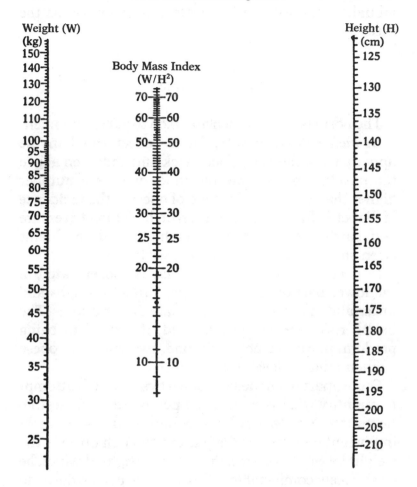

The index lies on the straight line drawn
from weight to height of an individual.

The distribution of fat within the body is an indication of the risk presented by the obesity of an individual. This distribution pattern is expressed as the ratio :

$$\frac{\text{Waist measurement at the navel}}{\text{Hip measurement}}$$

The norm is 0.85 for men and 0.65 to 0.85 for women.

In *male-pattern* obesity, fat is concentrated in the upper part of the body (face, neck and abdomen above the navel). In this case the index will be a number higher than 1. With this type of obesity, the incidence of diabetes, high blood cholesterol, high blood pressure and cardiovascular disease is high, with problems often showing up at a relatively early age.

In *female-pattern* obesity, the fat is concentrated in the lower part of the body (hips, buttocks, thighs and lower abdomen), the typical female distribution. The health risks are less pronounced, the problem being predominantly an aesthetic one, especially as obese women tend to develop cellulite.

Quite apart from medical statistics — which attempt to quantify what is more often perceived as an aesthetic matter or a sense of " not feeling right " — the most important concept for the patient to latch on to is the weight he would like to achieve, the weight at which he or she feels comfortable... this is what comes down to the " right " weight for that person, and that is the weight to be aimed for.

It may sometimes be a little above the theoretical norms, but why be more demanding than the overweight person is on his or her own account ? A target weight which the subject feels is a realistic goal is a better one to aim for than some theoretical norm laid down by medical opinion, which may simply leave the would-be slimmer discouraged by the apparent enormity of the task.

Conversely, it is no good for a woman to be brainwashed by the images peddled by the media and to set her sights on some mythical and unrealistic weight, which represents a quite unjustified aspiration and which her body, with its own very reasonable self-regulating mechanisms, will simply never accept.

A person's ideal weight, if such a thing there be, must be the product of careful evaluation and possibly the subject of a searching discussion between the overweight person and his or her doctor.

CONCLUSION

I hope that this book will have answered some of the questions that may have been in your mind. In any case, I hope you have enjoyed reading it.

It was certainly a great pleasure for me to write. Having to organise the material I had researched helped me to clarify details in my own mind and to deal systematically with information I had acquired piecemeal over the years.

In my researches and in putting the book together, I have become more and more confirmed in my conviction that " *we are what we eat!* "

In other words, the physical resources we have, or have left, our health and our life expectancy, are the direct legacy of how we have eaten in the past. I can assure you — but I am sure you no longer need convincing — that our *fitness, vitality, efficiency and dynamism depend directly on our eating habits.*

If you can learn to manage your eating, you will indeed have learnt to manage your life.

Modern man is, unfortunately, no longer a very

sensible being; he has lost sight of what constitutes true wisdom. He is capable of walking on the moon, but is no longer able to manage his own diet wisely.

One of the main tasks of a zoo-keeper is to take care of the animals' diet, for he knows that this is the key to the survival of species.

If a monkey ceases to be fertile, if a bear is losing its fur, if a lion is becoming too docile or if an elephant is losing its memory, the zoo-keeper's first reaction is to check the animal's diet and adjust it as appropriate.

But when the common man on the brink of the twenty-first century discovers, on getting up one morning, that he has spots all over his face, a crashing headache or foul-smelling breath, the doctor he consults will not even bother to question him on his eating habits. It is a splendid way to tackle problems in animals or machines but not, it seems, in people.

If a petrol-pump attendant puts diesel in your BMW by mistake, you will probably hit the roof, because you know what kind of fuel your car needs.

If you served an entrecôte steak to a giraffe, there is every probability the giraffe would ignore it, even if the animal had not eaten for a week. Animals have a sure instinct for what does not suit their metabolism. But man, this so-called " higher " mammal, endowed with intellect and articulate language, is the only living creature which will eat anything, or almost anything, without reflection and without the slightest reluctance or distaste.

The eating habits which have taken over in industrialised countries over the past few decades ought long since to have become a subject of concern for the governments of these countries.

A while ago I visited Disney World in Florida and, as I stood in the middle of the crowds which represented a cross-section of the American population, I again experienced a feeling of profound horror at the number of overweight people I could see around me. Something like 18 % of Americans, almost one in five, are either obese or well on their way to becoming obese.

Indeed, in the United States, obesity has become such a common social phenomenon that has become an accepted part of normal life. It is sobering to reflect that there is a connection between this and the fact that at Disney World there are as many wheelchairs as pushchairs available for the use of the visiting public.

The most powerful nation in the world is, paradoxically, truly on the road to physical degeneration. If this is the price of progress, it gives pause for thought.

All too few are those experts who point out that the phenomenon stems from a kind of mass intoxication arising out of the consumption of bad carbohydrates and excessive quantities of fats. What is most worrying of all in the United States is that obesity is disproportionately common among young people. This shows that the problem is linked to the deplorable eating habits which have proliferated since the Second World War.

Thank goodness we have not yet reached this point in France. I believe we have a good chance of not succumbing to the worst of the problem, given our cultural background and culinary tradition.

However, embryonic though it may still be in France, the phenomenon is present and growing. You have only to see the impressive numbers of fast food outlets which have sprung up in French cities in recent years. Moreover, when you look at the rising curve of the national statistics for soft drink consumption, there is every reason to suppose that the process of mass intoxication is under way even in France.

By giving in to advertising and laziness, we are unwittingly encouraging our children to adopt eating habits we do not find acceptable for ourselves. In a few years' time, it may be too late for remedial action.

There are those who can give you a detailed plan for getting 125,000 miles out of a car engine. But what could they be doing to increase the life expectancy of their children? The tragedy is that they do not even see it as cause for concern.

The human body is an amazing " machine ", capable of tolerating such excesses of treatment that people never realise when they are on the point of pushing it into the " danger zone ".

Women are a little less at risk than men, as they are endowed with greater sensitivity. By this, I mean they are more likely to react physically to stresses imposed on their body. This helps them throughout their lives to regulate their behaviour more sensibly and to pay attention to their body's needs.

Men, just because they are men, are less inclined to be aware of where their limitations lie. They tend to keep tugging as hard as they can at the rope for just as long as it does not snap. They will endure, rock-like, all the punishment they can heap upon themselves. But then one day, like the idol with the feet of clay, they will crack up.

All the nutritional mistakes you have made since childhood have been recorded by your body, which, on

226

every occasion, has taken appropriate measures to counteract them.

Often you will have experienced the side-effects of these " measures ", in the form of a variety of symptoms (headaches, gastric problems, intestinal trouble...)

These were warning signs that your body had had enough of your mistakes. They were also signs that its defences were being weakened and that your body was showing increasing sensitivity.

The particular problems, and therefore the symptoms, will vary from one individual to another. But the root cause is always the same : inadequate dietary management.

However, you have every right to feel cheered, because you are fortunate in your misfortune. By that I mean that by seeking a solution to a weight problem, you may also have hit upon a way of resolving all the other problems you have been suffering from.

This is just what happened to me a few years ago.

When I was a student, I was enrolled at an institute which prepared people for careers in the higher reaches of administration, or even politics (though this is not what I chose to do).

On the first day of term, the director addressed us all as follows :

" As Director of this Institute, my sole ambition during your course will be *to teach you how to read, write and speak.* "

As the author of this book, my sole ambition has been *to teach you how to eat.*

APPENDICES

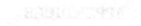

APPENDICE I

LIST OF PERMITTED FOODS
PHASE I : WEIGHT LOSS

STARTERS	MAIN COURSE	VEGETABLES/ SALADS	DESSERTS
EGGS	MEAT	TOMATOES	YOGURT
UNSMOKED HAM	(except liver)	SPINACH	CHEESE
SALADS	COOKED MEATS	CHICORY	Desserts based
TOMATO	FISH (all)	LETTUCE	on EGG CUSTARDS
- FRENCH BEANS	POULTRY	CRESS	
- CHICORY	RABBIT	LAMB'S LETTUCE	
- CUCUMBER	LOBSTER	DANDELION	
- CAULIFLOWER	EGGS	AUBERGINES	
RADISHES		CELERY	
LEEKS	DRESSINGS	CABBAGE	
LETTUCE, etc.		CAULIFLOWER	
CELERY	BUTTER	SAUERKRAUT	
MUSHROOMS	OLIVE OIL	FRENCH BEANS	
ASPARAGUS	PEANUT OIL	TURNIPS	
SMOKED SALMON	MARGARINE	LEEKS	
TUNA	MAYONNAISE	PEPPERS	
FRESH SALMON	BÉARNAISE SAUCE	COURGETTES	
SARDINES	SALT, PEPPER	BROCCOLI	
MUSSELS	ONIONS, GARLIC	FENNEL	
CRAB	SHALLOTS	SORREL	
LOBSTER	HERBS	MUSHROOMS	
		etc.	

NB : To make best use of this list, read the text of Chapter V on Phase I closely.
Beware of forbidden « PARASITES » (such as rice, sweetcorn or croutons)
which may be lurking in salads.
Beware too of eating too many cooked meats, cheeses and meats if you have
cholesterol problems.
All desserts are made with an artificial sweetener rather than sugar.

APPENDICE II

LIST OF PERMITTED FOODS
PHASE II : MAINTAINING A STABLE WEIGHT

STARTERS	MAIN COURSE	VEGETABLES/ SALADS	DESSERTS
FOIE GRAS *	MEAT (all)	TOMATOES	RASPBERRIES *
EGGS	COOKED MEATS	SPINACH	STRAWBERRIES *
COOKED MEATS *	FISH (all)	CHICORY	MELON
SALADS :	POULTRY	LETTUCE	YOGURT
- TOMATO	RABBIT	CRESS	FROMAGE FRAIS
- FRENCH BEANS	LOBSTER	LAMB'S LETTUCE	CHEESES
- CHICORY	EGGS	DANDELION	COAT'S CHEESES *
- WALNUTS		AUBERGINE	CANTAL CHEESE *
- CUCUMBER	DRESSINGS	CELERY	
- CAULIFLOWER		CABBAGE	BAVAROIS *
- MUSHROOMS	BUTTER	CAULIFLOWER	CHARLOTTE *
RADISHES	OLIVE OIL	SAUERKRAUT	CHOCOLATE
LEEKS	PEANUT OIL	FRENCH BEANS	MOUSSE *
LETTUCE	MARGARINE	TURNIPS	SORBETS *
CELERY	MAYONNAISE	LEEKS	GRATIN :
HEARTS OF PALM *	BÉARNAISE SAUCE	PEPPERS	- RASPBERRY
AVOCADO *	SALT	COURGETTES	- STRAWBERRY
TUNA	PEPPER	BROCCOLI	- BLACKBERRY
FRESH SALMON	MUSTARD *	FENNEL	- REDCURRANT
SMOKED SALMON	ONIONS	SORREL	
SARDINES	GARLIC	MUSHROOMS	
MUSSELS	SHALLOTS	SALSIFI	
CRAB	HERBS	LENTILS	
PRAWNS		BROAD BEANS	
SCAMPI		PEAS	
LOBSTER		DRIED BEANS	
OYSTERS *		CHICKPEAS	
SCALLOPS *			

NB : Foods marked with an asterisk are permitted in moderation.

233

APPENDIX 3

CHOCOLATE RECIPES
(FOR PHASE II)

CHOCOLATE MOUSSE

Makes 6 to 8 servings.

Ingredients

- 400g quality dark chocolate (containing 60-70 % cocoa)
- 8 eggs
- 7cl (half a glass) rum
- 1 orange
- 4 teaspoons instant coffee
- pinch of salt

Equipment

- Electric mixer/whisk
- Large saucepan

— Grater
— 2 large bowls
— Spatula

Break the chocolate into squares and place in the saucepan. Make half a cup of very strong coffee and add it to the chocolate. Add the rum. Melt the chocolate, either in a bain-marie or over very low heat. Stir with the spatula to make sure ingredients are mixed smoothly. If the mixture seems very thick, add a little water.
While the chocolate is melting, grate the orange rind, making sure to include no pith. Add half the orange zest to the mixture and stir. Break and separate the eggs, putting the yolks and whites into separate bowls. Beat the eggs whites with a pinch of salt until they are very stiff.

Add the chocolate mixture to the egg yolks and stir well until very smooth. Fold this mixture into the beaten egg whites until it is completely smooth, making sure there are no unmixed traces of either chocolate or egg white left at the bottom of the bowl.

You can either leave the mousse in the bowl (wiping the edges) or turn it into a large fruit-bowl. Before putting it in the refrigerator, sprinkle the remainder of the orange zest on top.

The mousse should be chilled for at least five hours before serving. Ideally, make it the day before.

BITTER CHOCOLATE FONDANT

Ingredients

— 400g quality dark chocolate (containing 60-70 % cocoa)
— 300g butter
— 5-7cl cognac
— 7 eggs
— 1 orange (optional)
— 4 teaspoons instant coffee
— 50g flour[1]

Equipment

— Electric mixer/whisk
— Large saucepan
— Loaf tin
— Grater
— Spatula
— Large bowl

Break the chocolate into squares and put them in the saucepan. Make half a cup of very strong coffee and add it to the chocolate. Add the cognac. Cut the butter into cubes and add to ingredients in the saucepan. Use a bain-marie or very low heat to melt

---

1. In relation to the total weight of the cake (about 1kg), 50g flour only accounts for a 5 % carbohydrate content, which is negligeable.

the chocolate and butter, stirring with the spatula until the mixture is smooth and creamy.

Break the eggs into the bowl and beat them, adding the flour a little at a time. Make sure there are no lumps.

Grate the orange peel and add half to the mixture in the saucepan. (The orange is optional. The combination of flavours is superb, but if you do not like orange flavoured chocolate, you can leave it out. If you do include the orange zest, do so in moderation and be careful to see it is quite free of pith.)

For preference use a non-stick mould. If your mould is on the small side (the cake rises in volume by 20 % during cooking), use some aluminium foil, well-greased with melted butter, to line the sides, making sure it comes well above the rim.

Add the lukewarm contents of the saucepan to the beaten eggs and mix until the mixture is really smooth. Pour into the mould. Sprinkle with the remainder of the orange zest. Place in the oven at 150 degrees C for 35 minutes.

Leave to cool at room temperature for three to four hours.

Cut thin slices (not more than a centimetre thick) and place gently on individual plates to serve, with two or three spoonfuls of custard.

Custard in sachets is quick to make. But be warned : it contains sugar and starch.

A home-made custard is better; you can use sweetener instead of sugar.

One last piece of advice : if you put the remainder of the cake away in the refrigerator, take it out *at least 4 hours* before eating it, as the cold spoils its smooth, creamy consistency.

238

APPENDIX 4

FURTHER RECIPES

My aim here is not to give you an impressive list of recipes to support the theme of the book.

The way I have gone about my task is to set out for you in practical terms the dietary principles on which you should base your eating from now on if you are to achieve your objective.

If you want to reduce the Method to the barest essentials, you could say that it rests on six basic concepts :

1. The calorie theory is mistaken, so you must rid yourself of your preconceptions on the subject.

2. Your diet should be balanced not within one meal but over the course of several.

3. In order to lose weight, you must avoid combining certain incompatible foods (namely, carbohydrates and lipids).

4. You should eat more fibre.

5. You should give up " bad carbohydrates " and eat only " good carbohydrates ".

6. You should monitor your fat consumption

closely, choosing "good lipids" in order to protect yourself against cardiovascular disease.

If you stick to the spirit of these principles, you will find it easy to plan each meal, whether at home or in a restaurant, and to select recipes from any convenient cookbook. So in this chapter you will just find a few examples of suitable recipes. From then on it is up to you to make your own choices.

WHOLEGRAIN RICE WITH TOMATO

Serves 4

— 1kg tomatoes (or a large tin of whole tomatoes)
— 3 or 4 large onions
— 250g wholegrain rice

Chop the onions very finely and cook gently in a little olive oil or margarine. Chop the tomatoes and reduce them in a large pan.

When the onions are browned, add them to the tomatoes. Continue cooking gently until reduced to a fairly thick sauce.

Meanwhile, boil the rice in salted water for about an hour and a quarter, just like ordinary rice. Serve either mixed with the tomato sauce or separately.

This rice dish could constitute in itself the main course of a meal. It could be preceded by a good vegetable soup. Be careful with the dessert though : if you want to eat cheese, it will have to be " very low fat " fromage frais, or you can eat " very low fat " yogurt. The only fruits you are allowed are strawberries or raspberries.

AUBERGINE GRATIN

Serves 6

— 4 or 5 good-sized aubergines
— 500g sausage meat
— 500g tomatoes
— 200g grated gruyère
— olive oil
— tarragon

Dice the aubergines and place in one or two pans. Sprinkle lightly with olive oil and cook over a low heat, stirring continuously to ensure they are evenly cooked.

When they have changed colour, season with salt and pepper and place in a large ovenproof dish. Bake for 40 minutes at about 150 degrees C.

Meanwhile, reduce the tomatoes as in the previous recipe. Separately, cook the sausage meat, stirring to separate it out.

When the aubergines are almost cooked, add the sausage meat and the tomato sauce and mix well. Spread the grated cheese on top and sprinkle with tarragon. Bake for a further 15 minutes under a medium grill.

Aubergine gratin is, again, a dish which can serve as the main course of a meal. As it contains meat (lipid-protein), it can be followed by cheese or other milk products.

Avoid fruit unless it is melon or strawberries.

The next two recipes are a little more sophisticated

but just as easy to make. They are good examples of what is known as " nouvelle cuisine ", and simple to make at home. They are wonderful served as starters at a rather special meal, such as for entertaining guests or a family celebration.

TUNA BAKE WITH LEEK COULIS

Serves 4 to 6

— 200g tin tuna in brine
— 200g crème fraîche
— 4 eggs
— 2 tablespoons chopped parsley

For the coulis :

— white part of 4 leeks
— 200g crème fraîche
— 20g butter
— salt and pepper

Preheat oven to 180 degrees C (gas mark 7). Butter a loaf tin.

Process the drained tuna and add the beaten eggs, crème fraîche, salt, pepper and parsley.

Turn the mixture into the loaf tin and place in the oven in a bain-marie for 35 minutes.

To make the leek coulis :

Wash the leeks and place the white parts in a pan. Season with salt and pepper, cover and sweat with a little butter over low heat for 20 minutes. Liquidise. Add the crème fraîche. Prior to serving reheat very gently.

Turn out the loaf and serve hot with the coulis.

Note : For a change, you can replace the tuna with salmon.

MONKFISH PATE

Serves 5

— 1kg monkfish (200g per person)
— 6 eggs
— small tin tomato puree
— 2 lemons

Cook the fish gently for about 20 minutes in a court-bouillon, waiting until the liquid is just simmering before adding the fish. Add the juice and zest of the two lemons while it is cooking.

Drain the fish, pressing out all the liquid with your hands. Remove the central bone. Place the fish in a well-buttered loaf tin or soufflé dish.

Lightly beat the eggs. Add the tomato puree, season with salt and pepper and pour the mixture over the fish.

Bake in a moderate oven (150 degrees C) for thirty minutes.

Turn out and serve cold with mayonnaise. To " give volume " to the mayonnaise, mix in a stiffly beaten egg white.

Note : This dish can be prepared the previous day. It should be chilled in the refrigerator for at least half a day before serving.

FLOUR-FREE SOUFFLE

Serves 4 to 5

— 300g " very low fat " fromage frais
— 150g grated gruyère
— 4 egg yolks
— 4 stiffly beaten egg whites
— salt and pepper

Mix together the fromage frais, grated gruyère and egg yolks.   Season with salt and pepper.

Beat the egg whites until they are really stiff.   Fold the two mixtures together and place in a soufflé dish at least 20cm across.

Cook in a hot oven (225 degrees C or Mark 7) for 30 to 40 minutes. Eat at once

Variant :   You can add to the first mixture 100g of lean ham or 115g pureed mushrooms.

STUFFED TOMATOES
(Also suitable for aubergines, courgettes, peppers, etc.)

Serves 4 to 5

— 6 good-sized tomatoes
— 400g sausage meat
— 300g mushrooms
— 1 onion
— salt and pepper
— optional : garlic and parsley

Cook the sausage meat in a frying-pan, seasoning if you like. Chop the onion and puree it. Wash the mushrooms and puree them too.

Mix the onion and mushroom purees. Lightly grease a pan with olive oil and heat the puree over a low heat, adding just a little salt.

Halve the tomatoes and place in a lightly oiled ovenproof dish. Bake in a hot oven for 30 minutes. Thoroughly mix the sausage meat and two thirds of the puree. Divide the mixture between the cooked tomatoes. Use the remaining third of the puree to put on top of the tomatoes, as if it were breadcrumbs. If you like, you can add the garlic and parsley, finely chopped.

Place in a very hot oven for 30 to 40 minutes. The dish can be placed under the grill, but not too closely or it will burn.

MOUSSAKA

Serves 6

— 2kg medium-sized aubergines
— 1 large onion, thinly sliced
— 1kg minced beef or lamb
— Half glass white wine
— 1kg tomatoes, peeled and chopped
— 3 tablespoons gruyère cheese, grated
— chopped parsley
— olive oil

Slice the aubergines thinly, sprinkle with salt and set aside for 1 hour.

Soften the onion by heating gently in 2 tablespoons of olive oil. Add the minced meat, separating the meat out as it cooks.

Add the tomatoes, wine and parsley. Season with salt and pepper. Leave to simmer for about 45 minutes.

Rinse and dry the aubergines. Fry gently on both sides in olive oil.

Grease an ovenproof dish and fill it with alternate layers of aubergine and the mince and tomato mixture.

Sprinkle with grated cheese and cook in a moderate oven for 45 minutes.

TUNA MOUSSE

Serves 6 to 8

— 100g " very low fat " fromage frais
— 400g tin tuna in brine
— 1 sachet gelatine
— 25cl white wine
— 1 spoon virgin olive oil
— 1 tablespoon vinegar
— 1 tablespoon chopped parsley
— 1 level teaspoon salt
— pepper
— mustard

For the decoration :
— slices of hard-boiled egg
— slices of tomato
— lettuce, parsley

Make up the gelatine as directed on the packet, replacing the half-glass of water with white wine.

Drain and flake the tuna. You can use an electric mixer if you like.

Thoroughly mix the tuna, mustard, olive oil, parsley, salt, pepper and vinegar.

When the gelatine has cooled to room temperature (about half an hour), mix it with the tuna mixture and the fromage frais.

Pour into a loaf tin, lightly greased with olive oil. Leave to set for 2 to three hours in the refrigerator.

Turn out and serve on a bed of lettuce leaves.   Deco-
rate with tomato, hard-boiled egg and parsley.

Serve with a dressing of your choice, such as a green
herb sauce or mayonnaise.

CUCUMBER AND FROMAGE FRAIS LOAF

Serves 8

— 2 × 500g cucumbers
— 750g well-drained " very low fat " fromage frais
— 10 leaves gelatine
— juice of half a lemon
— 5cl water
— 1 onion, very finely chopped or processed
— quarter clove garlic, very finely grated
— salt, pepper, coriander

Grate the two cucumbers finely, retaining a quarter of one of them for decoration. Place in a sieve, sprinkle with salt and leave to drain for 40 minutes. Drain very thoroughly and press out excess moisture with kitchen paper.

Soften the gelatine in cold water and then dissolve gently over heat in the 50cl water.

Mix together the fromage frais, cucumber, melted gelatine, onion, lemon, garlic and seasoning.

Lightly grease a large loaf-tin with olive oil. Line with very thin slices of cucumber.

Pour the mixture into the tin. Cover with the remaining cucumber slices. Chill for at least two and a half hours.

Turn out carefully and complete the decoration with slices of tomato, lettuce leaves, etc.

Serve as it is or with a more or less spicy dressing, according to taste.

CAULIFLOWER LOAF

Serves 8 to 10

— 1 good-sized cauliflower
— 100g " very low fat " fromage frais
— Half glass skimmed milk (made up to very smooth, thick, creamy consistency from powder)
— 6 eggs
— salt and pepper

Cut up cauliflower and wash in water containing a little vinegar. Drain and plunge into boiling water. Season with salt and cook for 5 minutes. Drain.

Mash the cauliflower to a puree, using the food processor if you like. Mix with the fromage frais, milk, eggs, salt and pepper.

Knead the mixture well and then place in a buttered loaf-tin. Cook for about an hour in a bain-marie at 200 degrees C (gas mark 5/6).

Leave for 15 minutes before turning out. Serve with a tomato coulis. This dish can be eaten warm or at room temperature.

CHILLED STRAWBERRY MOULD WITH COULIS

Serves 8 to 10

— 500g strawberries
— 100g " very low fat " fromage frais
— 5 egg whites
— 2 tablespoons lemon juice
— 5/6 spoonfuls powdered sweetener

Liquidise the strawberries or crush them to a puree. Whip the egg whites until stiff.

Mix together the strawberry puree, egg whites, fromage frais and sweetener until they are quite well blended. Add the lemon juice and pour the mixture into an oiled mould.

Leave in the ice-box or freezer for about 6 or 7 hours. Remove half an hour before serving.

To turn out, dip the mould in lukewarm water. Serve with a coulis, decorating with strawberry halves.

For the coulis : Mix 300g strawberries, 2 tablespoons powdered sweetener and the juice of half a lemon.

RASPBERRY BAVAROIS with coulis

Serves 5 to 6

— 500g raspberries
— 4 egg yolks
— 30cl milk
— 6 tablespoons powdered sweetener
— 3 sheets gelatine

Soak the gelatine leaves in cold water.

Beat the egg yolks in a saucepan and add the milk. Heat over a low flame, allowing the mixture to thicken until it will coat the spatula. Remove from heat.

Blend the raspberries to a puree and add the sweetener. Drain the gelatine and dissolve in the hot custard. Mix the custard and the raspberry puree together.

Pour into a lightly greased mould and leave to set in the refrigerator for at least 12 hours.

Serve cold with the raspberry coulis.

For the coulis : Puree 300g raspberries, adding the juice of one lemon and 3 or 4 tablespoons sweetener.

BIBLIOGRAPHY

PROTEINS :

APFELBAUM M., FORRAT C., NILLUS P., *Diététique et nutrition*, Ed. Masson, 1989.

BRINGER J., RICHARD J. L., MIROUZE J., *Evaluation de l'état nutritionnel protéique*, Rev. Prat., 1985, 35, 3, 17-22.

RUASSE J. P., *Les composants de la matière vivante*, Ed. L'indispensable en nutrition, 1988.

RUASSE J. P., *Des protides, pourquoi, combien ?* Ed. L'indispensable en nutrition, 1987.

CARBOHYDRATES :

BANTLE J. P., LAINE D. C., *Post prandial glucose and insulin responses to meals containing different carbohydrates in normal and diabetic subjects.* New Engl. J. Med. 1983, 309, 7-12.

BORNET F., *Place des glucides simples et des produits amylacés dans l'alimentation des diabétiques en 1985.* Fondation RONAC. Paris.

CRAPO P. A., *Plasma glucose and insulin responses to orally administrated simple and complex carbohydrates* Diabetes 1976, 25, 741-747.

CRAPO P. A., *Post prandial plasma glucose and insulin response to different complex carbohydrates.* Diabetes 1977, 26, 1178-1183.

CRAPO P. A., *Comparaison of serum glucose-insulin and glucagon responses to different types of carbohydrates in non insulin dependant diabetic patients,* Am. J. Clin. Nutr. 1981, 34, 84-90.

CHEW I., *Application of glycemic index to mixed meals.* Am. J. Clin. Nutr. 1988, 47, 53-56.

DANQUECHIN-DORVAL E., *Rôle de la phase gastrique de la digestion sur la biodisponibilité des hydrates de carbone et leurs effets métaboliques.* Journées de diabétologie de l'Hôtel-Dieu, 1975.

DESJEUX J. F., *Glycémie, insuline et acides gras dans le plasma d'adolescents sains après ingestion de bananes.*

255

Med. et Nutr. 1982, 18, 2, 127-30.

FEWKES D. W., *Sucrose* Science Progres, 1971, 59, 25, 39.

GABREAU T., LEBLANC H., *Les modifications de la vitesse d'absorption des glucides*, Med. et Nutr. 1983, XIX, 6, 447-449.

GUILLAUSSEAU P. J., GUILLAUSSEAU-SCHOLER, C., *Effet hyperglycémiant des aliments*, Gaz. Med. Fr. 1989, 96, 30, 61-63.

HEATON K. W., *Particule size of wheat, maïze and oat test meals : effects on plasma glucose and insulin responses and on the rate of starch digestion in vitro*, Am. J. Clin. Nutr. 1988, 47, 675-682.

HERAUD G., *Glucides simples, glucides complexes.*

HODORA D., *Glucides simples, glucides complexes et glucides indigestibles*, Gaz. Med. Fr. 1981, 88, 37, 5, 255-259.

JENKINS D. J. A., *Glycemic index of foods : a physiological basis for carbohydrates exchange*, Am. J. ; Clin. Nutr. 1981, 34, 362-366.

JENKINS D. J. A., *Dietary carbohydrates and their glycemic responses*, J.A.M.A. 1984, 2, 388-391.

JENKINS D. J. A., *Wholemeal versus wholegrain breads : proportion of whole or cracked grains and the glycemic response.*
Br. Med. J. 1988, 297, 958-960.

JIAN R., *La vidange d'un repas ordinaire chez l'homme : étude par la méthode radio-isotopique.*
Nouv. Presse Med. 1979, 8, 667-671.

KERIN O'DEA, *Physical factor influencing post prandial glucose and insulin responses to starch*, AM. J. Clin. Nutr. 1980, 33, 760-765.

NOUROT J., *Relationship between the rate of gastric emptying and glucose insulin responses to starchy food in young healty adults.*
Am. J. Clin. Nutr. 1988, 48, 1035-1040.

NATHAN D., *Ice-cream in the diet of insulin-dependant diabetic patients* J.A.M.A. 1984, 251, 21, 2825-2827.

NICOLAIDIS S., *Mode d'action des substances de goût sucré sur le métabolisme et sur la prise alimentaire. Les sucres dans l'alimentation.*
Cool. Sc. Fond. Fr ; Nutr. 1981.

O'DONNEL L. J. D., *Slze of flour particles and its relation to glycemia, insulinoemia and calonic desease.*
Br. Med. J. 17 June 1984, 298, 115-116.

REAVEN C., *Effects of source of dietary carbohydrates on plasma glucose and insulin to test meals in normal subjets.*
Am. J. Clin. Nutr. 1980, 33, 1279-1283.

ROUX E., *Index glycémique* Gaz. Med. Fr. 1988, 95, 18, 77-78.

RUASSE J. P., *Des glucides, pourquoi, comment ?*
Collection « L'indispensable en nutrition » 1987.

SCHLIENGER J. L., *Signification d'une courbe d'hyperglycémie orale plate ; comparaison avec un repas d'épreuve.*
Nouv. Pr. Med. 1982, 52, 3856-3857.

SLAMA G., *Corrélation between the nature of amount of carbohydrates in intake and insulin delivery by the artificiel pancreas in 24 insulin-dependant diabetics* Diabetes 1981, 30, 101-105.

SLAMA G., *Sucrose taken during mixed meal has no additional hyperglyceamic action over isocaloric amouts of starch in well-controled diabetics* Lancet, 1984, 122-124.

STACH J. K., *Contribution à l'étude d'une diététique rationnelle du diabétique : rythme circadien de la tolérance au glucose, intérêt du pain complet, intérêt du sorbitol.* Thèse pour le doctorat en Médecine, Cacn 1974.

THOBURN A. W., *The glyceemic index of food* Med. J. Austr. May 26 th 198 ?
144, 580-582.
VAGUE P., *Inflence comparée des différents glucides alimentaires sur la
sécrétion hormonale. Les sucres dans l'alimentation.* Collection Scientifi-
que de la Fondation Française pour la Nutrition.

LIPIDS :

BOURRE J. M., DURAND G., *The importance of dietary linoleic acid in
composition of nervous membranes.*
Diet and life style, new technology De M. F. Mayol 1988 John Libbey
Eurotext Ldt p. 477-481.
DYERBERG J., *Linolenic acid and eicospentaenoic acid* Lancet 26 janvier
1980, p. 199.
JACOTOT B., *Olive oil and the lipoprotein metabolism.* Rev. Fr. des Corps Gras,
1988, 2, 51-55.
MAILLARD C., *Graisses grises* Gazette Med. de Fr. 1989, 96, n° 22.
RUASSE J. P., *Des lipides, pourquoi, comment ?* Coll. L'Indispensable en
Nutrition.
VLES R. O., *Connaissances récentes sur les effets physiologiques* des margari-
nes riches en acide linoléique. Rev. Fr. des Corps Gras, 1980, 3, 115-120.

FIBRE :

« Concil Scientific Affairs », *Fibres alimentaires et santé* JAMA, 1984, 14, 190,
1037-1046.
ANDERSON J. W., *Dietary fiber : diabetes and obesity* Am. J. Gastroenterology
1986, 81, 898-906.
BERNIER J. J., *Fibres alimentaires, motricité et absorption intestinale. Effets
sur l'hyperglycémie post-prandiale.*
Journée de Diabétologie Hôtel-Dieu, 1979, 269-273.
HABER G. B., *Depletion and disruption of dietary fibre. Effets on satiety,
plasma glucose and serum insulin.*
Lancet 1977, 2, 679-682.
HEATON K. W., *Food fiber as an obstacle to energuintake.*
Lancet 1973, 2, 1418-1421.
HEATON K. W., *Dietary fiber in perspective* Humon Clin. Nutr. 1983, 37c, 151-
170.
HOLT S., *Effect of gel fibre on gastric emptying and absorption of glucose and
paracetamol.*
Lancet 1979, March 24, 636-639.
JENKINS D. J. A., *Decrease in post-prandial insulin and glucose concentration
by guar an pectin* Ann. Int. Med. 1977. 86. 20-33.
JENKINS D. J. A., *Dietary fiber, fibre analogues and glucose tolerance :
importance of viscosity* Br Med. J. 1978, 1, 1392-1394.
LAURENT B., *Etudes récentes concernant les fibres alimentaires* Med. et Nutr.
1983, XIX, 2, 95-122.
MONNIER L., *Effets des fibres sur le métabolisme glucidique* Cah. Nutr. Diet.
1983, XVIII, 89-93.
NAUSS K. M., *Dietary fat and fiber : relationship to caloric intake body growth,
and colon carcinogenesis.*
Am. J. Clin. Nutr. 1987, 45, 243-251.
SAUTIER C., *Valeur alimentaire des algues spirulines chez l'homme.* Ann. Nutr.
Alim. 1975, 29, 517.

257

Sautier C., *Les algues en alimentation humaine*. Cah. Nutr. Diet. 1987, 6, 469-472.

CHOLESTEROL (GENERAL) :

Basdevant A., Traynard P. Y., *Hypercholestérolémie Symptômes*, 1988, n° 12.
Bruckert E., *Les dyslipidémies Impact Médecin ;* Dossier du Praticien n° 20, 1989.
Luc G., Douste-Blazy P., Fruchart J. C., *Le cholestérol, d'où vient-il ? Comment circule-t-il ? Où va-t-il ?* Rev. Prat. 1989, 39, 12, 1011-1017.
Polonowski J., *Régulation de l'absorption intestinale du cholestérol.* Cahiers Nutr. Diet. 1989, 1, 19-25.

LIPIDS AND CHOLESTEROL :

Consensus : *Conférence on lowering blood cholesterol to prevent heart disease* JAMA 1985, 253, 2080-2090.
Betteridge D. J., *High density lipoprotein and coronary heart disease* Brit. Med. J. 15 avril 1989, 974-975.
Durand G. and all *Effets comparés d'huiles végétales et d'huiles de poisson sur le cholestérol du rat.*
Med. et Nutr. 1985, XXI, N° 6, 391-406.
Dyerberg J. and all *Eicosapentaenoic acid and prevention of thrombosis and atherosclerosis ?* Lancet 1978, 2, 117-119.
Ernst E., Le Mignon D., *Les acides gras omega 3 et l'artériosclérose* CR de Ther. 1987, V, N° 56, 22-25.
Field C., *The influence of eggs upon plasma cholesterol levels* Nutr. Rev. 1983, 41, N° 9, 242-244.
Fossati P., Fermonc. *Huiles de poisson, intérêt nutritionnel et prévention de l'athéromatose* N.P.N. Med. 1988, VIII, 1-7.
Gennes de J. L., Turping, Trffert J., *Correction thérapeutique des hyperlipidémies idiopathiques héréditaires. Bilan d'une consultation diététique standardisée* Nouv. Press Med. 1973, 2, 2457-2464.
Grundy M. A., *Comparaison of monosatured fatty acids and carbohydrates for lowering plasma cholesterol.*
N. Engl. J. Med. 1986, 314, 745-749.
Hay C. R. M., *Effect of fich on platelet kinetics in patients with ischaemic heart disease* The Lancet 5 juin 1982, 1269-1272.
Krmhout D., Bosschieter E. B., Lezenne-Coulander C., *The inverse relation between fish consumption and 20 year mortality from coronary heart disease.*
New. Engl. J. Med. 1985, 312, 1205-1209.
Leaf A., Weberpc Cardiovascular effects of n-3 fatty acides New Engl. J. Med. 1988, 318, 549-557.
Lemarchal P., *Les acides gras polyinsaturés en Omega 3* cah. Nutr. Diet. 1985, XX, 2, 97-102.
Marinier E., *Place des acides gras polyinsaturés de la famille n-3 dans le traitement des dyslipoprotéinémies.*
Med. Dig. Nutr. 1986, 53, 14-16.
Marwick C., *What to to about dietary satured fats ?* JAMA 1989, 262, 453.
Phillipson and al *Reduction of plasma lipids, lipoproteins and apoproteins by ietery fish oils in patients with hypertriglyceridemia.*
New. Engl. J. Med 1985, 312, 1210-1216.

258

PICLET G., *Le poisson, aliment, composition, intérêt nutritionnel* Cah. Nutr. Diet. 1987, XXII, 317-336.
THORNGREN M., *Effect of 11 week increase in dietary eicosapentaenoïc acid on bleeding time, lipids and platelet aggregation.*
Lancet 28 nov. 1981, 1190-11.
TURPIN G., *Régimes et médicaments abaissant la cholestérolémie* Rev. du Prat. 1989, 39, 12, 1024-1029.
VLES R. O., *Les acides gras essentiels en physiologie cardio-vasculaire* Ann. Nutr. Alim. 1980, 34, 255-264.
WOODCOCK B. E., *Beneficial effect of fish oil on blood viscosity in peripheral vascular disease.*
Br. Med. J. Vol. 288 du 25 février 1984, p. 592-594.

DIETARY FIBRE AND HIGH BLOOD CHOLESTEROL :

ANDERSON J. W., *Dietary fiber, lipids and atherosclerosis* Am. J. Cardiol. 1987, 60, 17-22.
GIRAULT A., *Effets bénéfiques de la consommation de pommes sur le métabolisme lipidique chez l'homme.*
Entretiens de Bichat 28 septembre 1988.
LEMONNIER D., DOUCET C., FLAMENT C., *Effet du son et de la pectine sur les lipides sériques du rat.*
Cah. Nutr. Diet. 1983, XVIII, 2, 99.
RAUTUREAU J., COSTE T., KARSENTI P., *Effets des fibres alimentaires sur le métabolisme du cholestérol.*
Cah. Nutr. Diet. 1983, XVIII, 2, 84-88.
SABLE-AMPLIS R., SICART R., BARON A., *Influence des fibres de pomme sur les taux d'esters de cholestérol du foie, de l'intestin et de l'aorte* Cah. Nutr. Diet. 1983, XVII, 2, 97.
TAGLIAFFERRO V. and al *Moderate guar-gum addition to usual diet improves peripheral sensibility to insulin and lipaemic profile in NIDDM* Diabète et Métabolisme 1985, 11, 380-385.
TOGNARELLI M., *Guar-pasta : a new diet for obese subjetsB* Acta Diabet. Lat. 1986, 23, 77.
TROWELL H., *Dietary fiber and coronary heart disease* Europ. J. Clin. Biol. Res. 1972, 17, 345.
VAHOUNY G. U., *Dietary fiber, lipid metabolism and atherosclerosis* Fed. Proc. 1982, 41, 2801-2806.
ZAVOLAL J. H., *Effets hypolipémiques d'aliments contenant du caroube* Am. J. Clin. Nutr. 1983, 38, 285-294.

VITAMINS, TRACE ELEMENTS AND HIGH BLOOD CHOLESTEROL :

1) Vitamin « E »
CAREW T. E., *Antiatherogenic effect of probucol unrelated to ist hypocholesterolemic effect* P.N.A.S.
USA June 1984, Vol. 84, p. 7725-7729.
FRUCHART J. C., *Influence de la qualité des LD sur leur métabolisme et leur athérogénicité (inédit).*
JURGENS G., *Modification of human serum LDL by oxydation* Chemistry and Physics of lipids 1987, 45, 315-336.
STREINBRECHER V. P., *Modifications of LDL by endothelial cells involves lipid peroxydation* P.N.A.S.
USA June 1984, Vol. 81, 3883-3887.

2) Selenium

LUOMA P. V., *Serum selenium, glutatione peroxidase, lipids, and human liver microsomal enzyme activity.*
Biological Trace Element Research 1985, 8, 2, 113-121.
MITCHINSON M. J., *Possible role of deficiency of selenium and vitamin E in atherosclerosis* J. Clin Pathol. 1984, 37, 7, 837.
SALONEN J. T., *Serum fatty acids, apolipoproteins, selenium and vitamin antioxydants and risk of death from coronary artery disease* Am. J. Cardiol. 1985, 56, 4, 226-231.

3) Chromium

ABRAHAM A. S., *The effect of chromiuon established atherosclerotic plaques in rabbits* Am. J. Clin. Nutr. 1980, 33, 2294-2298.
GORDON T., *High density lipoprotein as a protective factor against coronary heart disease.*
The Framingham study Am. J. Med. 1977, 62, 707.
OFFENBACHER E. G., *Effect of chromium-rich yeast on glucose tolerance a blood lipids in elderly subjets* Diabetes 1980, 29, 919-925.

COFFEE AND HIGH BLOOD CHOLESTEROL :

ARNESEN E., *Coffe and serum cholesterol* Br. Med. J. 1984, 288, 1960.
HERBERT P. N., *Caffeine does not affect lipoprotein metabolism.* Clin. Res. 1987, 35, 578A.
HILL C., *Coffe consumption and cholesterol concentration.* Letter to editor Br. Med. J. 1985, 290, 1590.
THELLE D. S., *Coffe and cholesterol in epidemiological and experimental studies.* Atherosclerosis 1987, 67, 97-103.
THELLE D. S., *The Tromso Heart Study. Does coffe raise serum cholesterol?* N. Engl. J. Med. 1983, 308, 1454-1457.

THE CALORIE MYTH :

ASTIER-DUMAS M., *Densité calorique, densité nutritionnelle, repères pour le choix des aliments* Med. Nutr. 1984, XX, 4, 229-234.
BELLISLE F., *Obesity and food intake in children : evidence for a role of metabolic andlor behavioral daily rythms.*
Appetite 1988, 11, 111-118.
BROWNELL K. D., *The effects of repeated cycles of weight loss and regain in rats* Phys. Behavior 1986, 38, 459-464.
HERAUD G., *Densité nutritionnelle des aliments* Gaz. Med. FR. 1988, 95, 13, 39-42.
LEIBEL R. J., *Diminished energy requirements in reduced obese persons* Metabolism 1984, 33, 164-170.
ROLLAND-CACHERA M. F., BELLISLEF. *No correlation beetween adiposity and food intake : why are working class children fatter?*
Am. J. Clin. Nutr. 1986, 44, 779-787.
ROLAND-CACHERA M. F., DEHEEGER M., *Adiposity and food intake in yong children : the environmental challenge to individual susceptibility* Br. Med. J. 1988, 296, 1037-1038.
RUASSE J. P., *des calories, pourquoi? Combien?* Coll. L'indispensable en Nutrition 1987.
RUASSE J. P., *L'approche homéopathique du traitement des obésités*, Paris, 1988.

260

SPITZER L., RODIN J., *Human eating behavior : a critical review of studi in normal weight and overweight individuals* Appetite 1981, 2, 293.

LOUIS-SYLVESTRE J., *Poids accordéon : de plus en plus difficile à perdre* Le Gén. 1989, 1087, 18-20.

INSULIN :

BASDEVANT A., *Influence de la distribution de la masse grasse sur le risque vasculaire,* La Presse Médicale, 1987, 16, 4.

CLARK M. G., *Obesity with insulin resistance. Experimental insights.* Lancet, 1983, 2, 1236-1240.

FROMAN L. A., *Effect of vagotomy and vagal stimulation on insulin secretion.* Diabetes 1967, 16, 443-448.

GROSS P., *De l'obésité au diabète.* L'actualité diabétologique N° 13, p. 1-9.

GUY-GRAND B., *Variation des acides gras libres plasmatiques au cours des hyperglycémies provoquées par voie orale.* Journées de Diabétologie de l'Hôtel-Dieu, 1968, p. 319.

GUY-GRAND B., *Rôle éventuel du tissu adipeux dans l'insulino-résistance.* Journées de Diabétologie de l'Hôtel-Dieu, 1972, 81-92.

JEANRENAUD B., *Dysfonctionnement du système nerveux. Obésité et résistance à l'insuline.* M/S Médecine-Sciences 1987, 3, 403-410.

JEANRENAUD B., *Insulin and obesity* Diabetologia, 1979, 17, 135-138.

KOLTERMAN O. G., *Mechanisms of insulin resistance in human obesity. Evidence for receptor and post-receptor effects.* J. Clin. Invest. 1980, 65, 1272-1284.

LAMBERT A. E., *Enhancement by caffeine of glucagon-inducet and tolbutamide inducet insulin release from isolated fœtal pancreatic tissue* Lancet, 1967, 1, 819-820.

LAMBERT A. E., *Organocultures de pancréas fœtal de rat : étude morphologique et libération d'insuline in vitro.* Journées de Diabétologie de l'Hôtel-Dieu, 1969, 115-129.

LARSON B., *Abdominal adipose tissue distribution, obesity and risk of cardiovascular disease and death.* Br. Med. J. 1984, 288, 1401-1404.

LE MARCHAND-BRUSTEL Y., *Résistance à l'insuline dans l'obésité* M/S Médecine-Sciences 1987, 3, 394-402.

LINQUETTE C., *Précis d'endocrinologie,* Ed. Masson, 1973, p. 658-666.

LOUIS-SYLVESTRE J., *La phase céphalique de sécrétion d'insuline.* Diabète et métabolisme, 1987, 13, 63-73.

MARKS V., *Action de différents stimuli sur l'insulinosécrétion humaine : influence du tractus gastro-intestinal.* Journées de Diabétologie de l'Hôtel-Dieu, 1969, 179-190.

MARLISSE E. B., *Système nerveux central et glycorégulation.* Journées de Diabétologie de l'Hôtel-Dieu, 1975, 7-21.

MEYLAN M., *Metabolic factors in insulin resistance in human obesity.* Metabolism, 1987, 36, 256-261.

WOODS S. C., *Interaction entre l'insulinosécrétion et le système nerveux central.* Journées de Diabétologie de l'Hôtel-Dieu, 1983.

HYPOGLYCAEMIA :

CAHILL G. F., *A non editorial on non hypoglycemia* N. Engl. J. Med. 1974, 291, 905-906.

CATHELINEAU G., *Effect of calcium infusion on post reactive hypoglycemia* Horm. Meatb. Res. 1981, 13 ? 646-647.

CHILES R., *Excessive serum insulin response to oral glucose in obesity and mild diabets* Diabetes 1970, 19, 458.

CRAPO P. A., *The effects of oral fructose, cucrose and glucose in subjets with reactive hypoglycemia.* Diabetes care 1982, 5, 512-517.

DORNER M., *Les hypoglycémies fonctionnelles* Rev. Prat. 1972, 22, 25, 3427-3446.

FAJANS S. S., *Fasting hypoglycemia in adults* New Engl. J. Med. 1976, 294, 766-772.

FARRYKANT M., *The problem of fonctionnal hyperinsulinism of fonctional hypoglycemia attributed to nervous causes.* Metabolism 1971, 20, 6, 428-434.

FIELD J. B., *Studies on the mechanisms of ethanol induced hypoglycemia* J. Clin. Inverst. 1963, 42, 497-506.

FREINKEL N., *Alcohol hypoglycemia* J. Clin. Invest. 1963, 42, 1112-1133.

HARRIS S., *Hyperinsulinism and dysinsulinism* J.A.M.A. 1924, 83, 729-733.

HAUTECOUVERTURE M., *Les hypoglycémies fonctionnelles* Rev. Prat. 1985, 35, 31, 1901-1907.

HOFELDT F. D., *Reactive hypoglycemia* Metab. 1975, 24, 1193-1208.

HOFELDT F. D., *Are abnormalities in insulin secretion responsable for reactive hypoglycemia ?* Diabetes 1974, 23, 589-596.

JENKINS D. J. A., *Decrease in post-prandial insulin and glucose concentrations by guar and pectin.* Ann. Intem. Med. 1977, 86, 20-23.

JOHNSON D. D., *Reactive hypoglycemia* J.A.M.A. 1980, 243, 1151-1155.

JUNG Y., *Reactive hypoglycemia in women* Diabetes 1971, 20, 428-434.

LEFEBVRE P., *Statement on post-prandial hypoglycemia* Diabetes care 1988, 11, 439-440.

LEFEBVRE P., *Le syndrome d'hypoglycémie réactionnelle, mythe ou réalité ?* Journées Annuelles de l'Hôtel-Dieu, 1983, 111-118.

LEICHTER S. B., *Alimentary hypoglycemia : a new appraisal* Amer. J. Nutr. 1979, 32, 2104-2114.

LEV-RAN A., *The diagnosis of post-prandial hypoglycemia* Diabetes 1981, 30, 996-999.

LUBETZKI J., *Physiopathologie des hypoglycémies* Rev. Prat. 1972, 22, 25, 3331-3347.

LUYCKY A. S., *Plasma insulin in reactive hypoglycemia* Diabetes 1971, 20, 435-442.

MONNIER L. H., *Restored synergistic entero-hormonal response after addition dietary fibre to patients with impaired glucose tolerance and reactive hypoglycemia* Diab. Metab. 1982, 8, 217-222.

O'KEEFE S. J. D., *Lunch time gin and tonic : a cause of reactive hypoglycemia* Lancet 1977, 1, June 18, 1286-1288.

PERRAULT M., *Le régime de fond des hypoglycémies fonctionnelles de l'adulte* Rev. Prat. 1963, 19, 4025-4030.

SENG G., *Mécanismes et conséquences des hypoglycémies* Rev. Prat. 1985, 35, 31, 1859-1866.

SERVICE J. F., *Hypoglycemia and the post-prandial syndrom* New Engl. J. Med. 1989, 321, 1472.

SUSSMAN K. E., *Plasma insulin levels during reactive hypoglycemia* Diabetes 1966, 15, 1-14.

TAMBURRANO G., *Increased insulin sensitivity in patients with idiopathic reactive hypoglycemia.*
J. Clin. Endocr. Metab. 1989, 69, 885.

TAYLOR S. I., *Hypoglycemia associated with antibodies to the insulin receptor.*
New Engl. J. Med. 1982, 307, 1422-1426.

YALOW R. S., *Dynamics of insulin secretion in hypoglycemia* Diabetes 1965, 14, 341-350.

CONTENTS

266

DINE OUT AND LOSE WEIGHT
by Michel Montignac

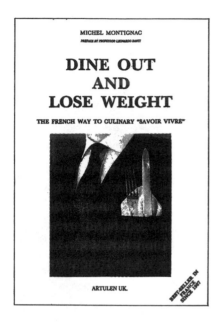

Michel Montignac has revolutionized France with his revelations on diet and nutrition. In his book, the former executive questions a number of preconceived ideas and established myths on how to lose weight.

This European bestseller will show you how to lose weight and continue to dine out. You will learn how to easily shed your surplus pounds without counting calories or restricting yourself to the point of starvation.

More importantly, you will learn how to stabilize your weight from now on, achieve top physical and mental well-being, and, from time to time, indulge in guilt-ridden pleasures. You will develop healthy eating habits that do not rule out wine or chocolate.

Montignac's method is recognized by French medical institutions. It has been adopted by celebrities, politicians and professional athletes. The author himself teaches his method in seminars that have attracted an international clientele.

This landmark in the history of nutritional sciences, fun and easy to read, is a savory antidote to "bland" meals and traditional diets. This book is an indispensable tool for every business man and woman, or any individual with an epicurean flair, who is determined to stay fit without abandoning the culinary pleasures of life.

It is dedicated to all gourmets with an appreciation for "savoir vivre".

ISBN 2-906236-17-9
298 pages. Format 18 × 27
Prix : £ 11,95

Distributor : Biblios Ltd.
Artulen UK 108 New Bond Street LONDON W1Y9AA

Restaurant Michel MONTIGNAC
« Le Pavillon Maillot »
7 rue Waldeck-Rousseau
75017 PARIS
Tél : (1) 45.72.39.41

MONTIGNAC FOOD BOUTIQUES OPERATE IN :

United-Kingdom :

160, Old Brompton Road LONDON SW5 OBA (*o)   Phone : (44) 071.370.2010

France :

1) 14, rue de Maubeuge 75009 PARIS   Phone : (1) 49.95.93.42
2) 5, rue Benjamin-Franklin 75116 PARIS   Phone : (1) 45.27.35.73

Belgium :

1351, Chaussée de Waterloo 1180 BRUXELLES   Phone : (32) 2.374.95.31

Guadeloupe :

25, Place de l'Église 97110 POINT-A-PITRE   Phone : (590) 93.21.76

Martinique :

77, rue de Blénac 97220 FORT-DE-FRANCE   Phone : (596) 70.21.69

Switzerland :

1) 48, rue de la Terrassière 1207 GENÈVE(*)   Phone : (41) 22.786.87.44
2) 19, rue Mauverney 1196 GLAND-VAUD   Phone : (41) 21.364.77.24

* Mail order facility available
o Catering

Reproduit et achevé d'imprimer
sur Roto-Page en octobre 1996
par l'Imprimerie Floch
à Mayenne
Dépôt légal : avril 1994
Numéro d'impression : 40437

Imprimé en France